Dissection on Display

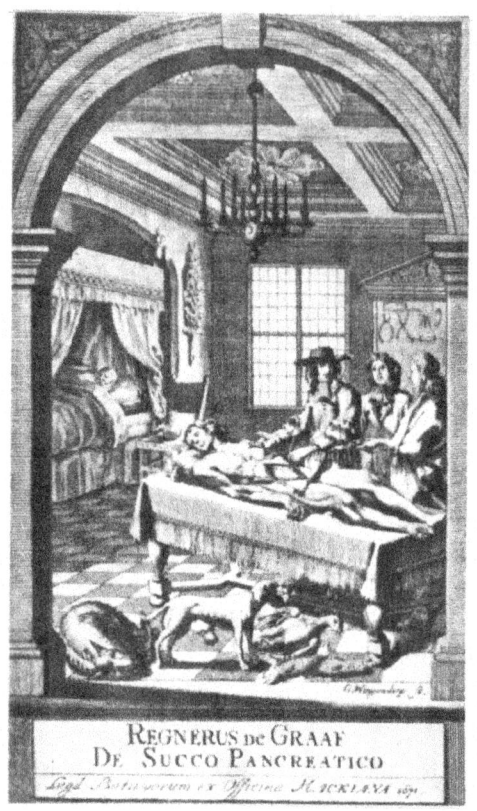

REGNERUS de GRAAF
DE SUCCO PANCREATICO

Dissection on Display
Cadavers, Anatomists and Public Spectacle

CHRISTINE QUIGLEY

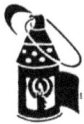

McFarland & Company, Inc., Publishers
Jefferson, North Carolina, and London

ALSO BY CHRISTINE QUIGLEY AND FROM MCFARLAND

Conjoined Twins: An Historical, Biological and Ethical Issues Encyclopedia (2003; paperback 2006)

Skulls and Skeletons: Human Bone Collections and Accumulations (2001; paperback 2008)

Modern Mummies: The Preservation of the Human Body in the Twentieth Century (1998; paperback 2006)

The Corpse: A History (1996; paperback 2005)

Death Dictionary: Over 5,500 Clinical, Legal, Literary and Vernacular Terms (compiled and edited by; 1994; paperback 2011)

Frontispiece: In this illustration, which appeared on the title page of his 1671 text on pancreatic secretions, Dutch surgeon Dr. Regnerus de Graaf stands before a dissecting table with two companions. In front of the table are several animals, including a live dog, and on the wall hang his surgical instruments. An ailing man lies in the bed on the left (*Wellcome Images*).

LIBRARY OF CONGRESS CATALOGUING-IN-PUBLICATION DATA

Quigley, Christine, 1963–
    Dissection on display : cadavers, anatomists and public spectacle / Christine Quigley.
       p.   cm.
    Includes bibliographical references and index.

ISBN 978-0-7864-4429-8
softcover : acid free paper ∞

1. Human dissection — History. I. Title.
QM33.4.Q44 2012
611—dc23   2012005443

BRITISH LIBRARY CATALOGUING DATA ARE AVAILABLE

© 2012 Christine Quigley. All rights reserved

No part of this book may be reproduced or transmitted in any form or by any means, electronic or mechanical, including photocopying or recording, or by any information storage and retrieval system, without permission in writing from the publisher.

On the cover: *Dissection before a group of students,* 17th c. (courtesy of the National Library of Medicine); background image © 2012 Shutterstock

Manufactured in the United States of America

McFarland & Company, Inc., Publishers
  Box 611, Jefferson, North Carolina 28640
    www.mcfarlandpub.com

Contents

ACKNOWLEDGMENTS	vii
PREFACE	1
DEFINITIONS OF DISSECTION AND AUTOPSY	9
DISSECTION CHRONOLOGY	13
INTRODUCTION	17

1. Anatomists as Procurers of Cadavers	35
• Alexander Monro Primus (1697–1767) and His Legacy	58
• John Hunter (1728–1793) and His Brother	64
• Sir Astley Cooper (1768–1841) and His Boast	70
2. Anatomists as Demonstrators and Educators	75
• Mondino de Liuzzi (c. 1270–1326) and His History	90
• Andreas Vesalius (1514–1564) and His Modernity	93
• John Bell (1763–1820) and His Illustrations	98
• Henry Gray (1827–1861) and His Textbook	101
3. Anatomists as Preparators and Collectors	105
• Frederik Ruysch (1638–1731) and His Assemblages	109
• William Cheselden (1688–1752) and the Skeleton	121
• Clemente Susini (1757–1814) and the Anatomical Waxes	125
• Honoré Fragonard (1732–1799) and His Preparations	138
4. Anatomists as Superlatives and Showmen	144
• Nicolaes Tulp (1593–1674) and His Fame	158
• Georges Cuvier (1769–1832) and His Venus	160
• Thomas Pettigrew (1791–1865) and His Mummies	166

Contents

- P.T. Barnum (1810–1891) and His Hoax   178
- Gunther von Hagens (1945–) and His Spectacles   180

CONCLUSION   197
BIBLIOGRAPHY   205
INDEX   215

Acknowledgments

This book could not have been written without the cooperation and support of my parents, Donna and Del Gritman and James Michael and Sarah Quigley, who relocated me from northern Virginia to central Florida and have ensured my continued comfort and productivity. Without naming names (because I am afraid I will inadvertently leave some out), I have received invaluable understanding and encouragement during my move and my writing from the rest of my family; my former colleagues at Georgetown University; my longstanding friends in the Washington, D.C., area; my new friends here in Florida; the dozens of like-minded individuals I have met worldwide through my research and my blog Quigley's Cabinet, some of whom I have had the pleasure of meeting in person; and the many teachers who have made an impression on me, in particular Samuel F. Pickering, Jr., of the University of Connecticut and James F. Schaefer, Jr., of Georgetown University. My thanks to Carrie Hoggan for confirming the location in Edinburgh of some of the souvenirs made from the skin of William Burke; to Gillian Scott, University of York, for sharing her unpublished work on mummy unrollings; and to Jeremy Knight, Curator & Heritage Officer, Horsham Museum, for relaying details about the dissection of Richard Grazemark. I am grateful also for permission to reprint from the image databases of the National Library of Medicine in Bethesda, Maryland, and the Wellcome Institute in London, and from the following institutions and individuals: Royal Picture Gallery Mauritshuis, The Hague, The Netherlands; Peter Nahum at the Leicester Galleries, London; Barry Iverson, Barry Iverson Photography, Cairo; Gert-Horst Schumacher, Universität Rostock, Mecklenburg-Vorpommern, Germany; St. Edmundsbury Borough Council, Suffolk, England; St. John's College,

ACKNOWLEDGMENTS

Cambridge, England; University of Pennsylvania Art Collection, Philadelphia; WeirdNJ.com, New Jersey; and Yale University, Harvey Cushing/John Hay Whitney Medical Library, New Haven, Connecticut.

Preface

On November 13, 2010, an assistant professor at Kankanwadi Ayurveda Medical College in Belgaum, Karnataka, India, took up a scalpel to demonstrate human anatomy for his medical students. The subject was an eighty-nine-year-old man by the name of B.S. Ramannavar who felt strongly about donating his body to science. He wanted his remains to be put to use rather than merely burned or buried, a sentiment that convinced several of his family members — including his wife and his daughter-in-law — to pledge to do the same. The slender body of the man who had been a freedom fighter and a dentist lay on the table, draped with a white sheet. The anatomist knew the body well, though he had not yet opened it. The man had specifically requested on his deathbed that the young professor anatomize his remains for the benefit of medical education and research. The professor had been inspired by this particular body bequest to start a charitable trust in the man's name, through which he has motivated more than one hundred people to pledge their bodies. The students leaned forward as Dr. Mahantesh B. Ramannavar motioned to them how he would make the first incision. The cadaver was his father.

The precedent for this event, which was unusual enough to be featured in the local media, dates back four hundred years. Seventeenth-century English anatomist William Harvey, best known for discovering the circulation of the blood, dissected the bodies of his father, his sister, and his cousin's husband. Although these anatomical dissections were conducted privately, Harvey mentioned them in his lectures to students, noting the huge size of the colon he removed from his father's abdomen and the heavy weight of his sister's spleen. Historian Lynda Payne (2002) writes, "Anatomical knowledge which raised a physician above his non-

Preface

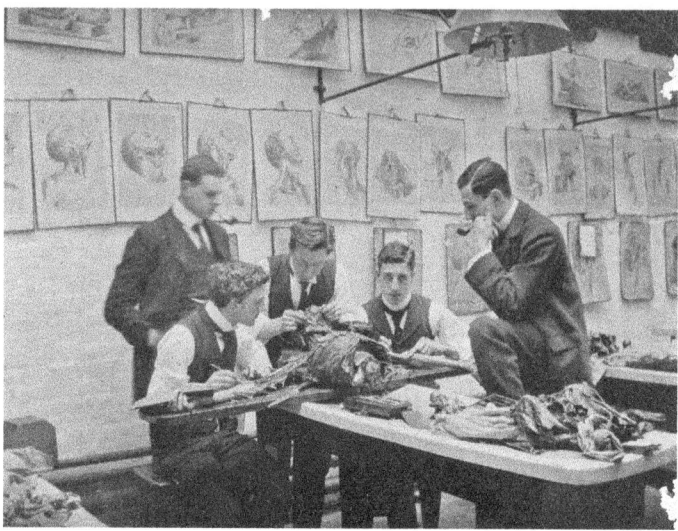

Two professors instruct three students (in rolled-up shirtsleeves) during a typical anatomical dissection in a windowless gas-lit room in the early 20th century. The bisected cadaver lies on the table and anatomical illustrations line the walls (*Wellcome Images*).

anatomically minded peers, while seeing and then constantly performing dissections and postmortems, allowed Harvey and his admirers to continually rehearse a certain emotionless response to suffering in living bodies. Yet these rehearsals were not often successful, for Harvey or his disciples. The activities of Harvey, his peers and followers did not escape the notice of the public and a particular stereotype emerged of a stoic, but flamboyant and deeply troubling, anatomist-physician. Critics of dissection-crazed medical men compared anatomy to the practice of cannibalism and suggested that those who frequently cut on the dead lost, or perhaps never even learned, a humane bedside manner toward the living." Anatomists have had a reputation as ghouls since the era when they were indebted to the hangman and the bodysnatcher for their subjects. That reputation continues in the present day, when the rare anatomist to step out of the sequestered medical school anatomy laboratory faces criticism for dabbling in corpses — particularly for doing so publicly.

The general public of today shuns the idea of watching the anatomist at work, a task that the people of previous generations, when they were allowed to observe, found both enlightening and entertaining. If you were present in Bologna in 1540, for instance, you may have seen visiting anatomist Andreas Vesalius throw off tradition, step down from his podium, and take up the scalpel himself to conduct the semi-annual comparative dissection of a human and an ape. Like the rest of the audience — consisting of faculty and physicians, medical students, and interested laypersons — you would have been spellbound as Vesalius performed the functions of three men in the temporary wooden theater. He lectured based on his own observations, rather than referring to an outdated textbook; he pointed out the structures he was discussing, sometimes making quick charcoal sketches to better explain their relationships to one another; and he exposed the interiors of man and animal to show how *dissimilar* they are. Watching a public dissection was truly an instructive experience, although you may have been both distracted by the crowd of two hundred and unaware of how revolutionary the renowned Belgian anatomist's methods and conclusions were.

Nearly two hundred years later, still in Italy, you would not have missed the lavish spectacle that was made of the annual dissection, which coincided with the celebration of carnival. The anatomy theater was lit with candles and the wood-paneled walls were decorated with damask for the occasion. A formal seating arrangement would have been drawn up to maintain the order of the noisy crowd of doctors, students, university and city employees, and ordinary citizens. Another benefit of attending the first and last lesson would be to see the most eminent Bolognese officials, but even in the two weeks in between, the daily event would attract dozens of attendees in their festival costumes. A hierarchy of professors would have taken up the demonstration of the cadaver's organs in turn, as masses were said elsewhere for the soul of the deceased. In provoking the audience with questions, the scholars may have been answered with indignities by unruly members of the crowd. The dissectors may even have had to guard the opened body from their grabbing hands. Despite such occasional disturbances of protocol, public dissection was a tradition, rich in ritual and ceremony, that had been carried on for generations.

Another tradition was that of the Grand Tour, in which well-to-do young adults embarked on a standard travel itinerary as a rite of passage.

Preface

If as a touring Englishman your itinerary had veered south of Paris, you may have found yourself in the anatomical cabinet of Honoré Fragonard at the veterinary school in Alfort. The sights you saw here had little in common with the girl on a swing in the familiar Rococo painting of his cousin. There was no billowy orange dress to cover the anatomized rider of a similarly anatomized horse. And if you had listened to rumor, you may be convinced that the man responsible for this monstrosity had dissected his own girlfriend before mounting her in the saddle. If your stop in Amsterdam had included the museum of Frederik Ruysch, you met with much smaller specimens — babies, in fact. But Ruysch was said to be a singular embalmer, and his anatomical preparations bore this out. The infants in the bottles were positively aglow. And even their detached limbs were trimmed with lace and other dainties. But how to describe to the family upon your return the strange little dioramas that the anatomist so cleverly prepared, with fetal skeletons weeping and playing the violin? It would be much easier to describe the anatomical wax models you went to see at La Specola in Florence. You might omit the fact that the figures were so sensually posed and describe how they were patterned after classical sculpture, suggesting to your listeners that wax's transparency and luminosity may just make it the perfect medium for portraying human flesh. You wouldn't have to tell them that one of the modelers had demonstrated how the "Venus" statue was in fact pregnant by pulling apart her abdomen to remove her womb and reveal its contents.

If you were one of the 20,000 citizens of Edinburgh who assembled on a rainy day in January 1829 to witness the execution of notorious bodysnatcher William Burke, you may have arrived early to secure a spot up front. Your audible cheer would have joined with others as workers finished assembling the wooden gibbet for the occasion. Perhaps you cheered again when the body of the murderer dropped in the noose. Hopefully the morbid sight did not distract you so much that you became prey to one of the pickpockets who were known to circulate in such crowds. Having read the handbill that had been posted about Burke's sentence, you were aware that he was to be dissected in addition to being hanged by the neck until dead. After watching the hangman cut down the body within an hour of having fulfilled his duty, you strained to see

Preface

the corpse handed off to the anatomists. But you may afterwards have felt slighted that the dissection was not, as you had hoped, open to the public. Instead, Burke's lifeless and unclothed body was anatomized before only a select group of students. You may have been disappointed enough to demand entrance with the rest of an unruly crowd that was finally allowed to file past the exposed corpse. You were glad to have the chance to see the vile man before the anatomist harvested his skeleton for the university museum. Only later did you learn that Burke's skin had been removed to be tanned and crafted into souvenirs, including wallets, but you did not feel the need to own such tangible evidence when the mere sights and sounds of the full punishment would not soon vanish from your memory. Observing the dissection of designated criminals was, after all, the right of an interested public.

As a Victorian interested in ancient Egypt, you would have been delighted to hold tickets to the 1843 public "unrolling" of a mummy. The honors were to be performed by renowned London surgeon Thomas Pettigrew. Entering Canterbury Theatre, you would have noticed that the orchestra pit had been boarded over to accommodate the capacity crowd and the walls had been decorated to match the Egyptian theme of the lecture. "Mummy" Pettigrew, as he was nicknamed in the popular press, held the audience's attention with his words for an hour. After this promising introduction, he and his son began unwrapping the preserved body of a young man. As they cut away the resinous linens, your nose may have wrinkled from the dust and odd odor that circulated in the air. You would have been mesmerized by the sight and sound of the skull being sawn open to reveal the pitch inside. As the unwrapped mummy was held up for the crowd, you would have shown your appreciation — like the others — with enthusiastic applause. Coming away from the theatre at eleven o'clock when the evening's program ended, you may have been unaware of the late hour as you fingered the bit of linen you had received as a souvenir. You turned it in your hand the following day as you read a glowing review of the event you were lucky enough to have attended in person. A public dissection such as this was an exotic entertainment and a moving and memorable experience.

Dissections have been practiced in many ways over the centuries — sometimes publicly, sometimes semi-privately — with the anatomist as impresario. Some of these anatomists have become very famous (John Hunter), and others of them remain relatively obscure to us (Henry Gray). Some have been immortalized in paintings by the masters (Nicolaes Tulp), and others are remembered by just a few vignettes of biographical material in classical sources (Mondino de Liuzzi). Some are associated with the grand spectacles of today (Gunther von Hagens), others with the envied technical proficiency of yesterday (Honoré Fragonard). Here is an attempt to make sense of the chronology the anatomists laid down, the relationships they had with one another, and the mindset they shared given their dubious history of patronizing bodysnatchers and brawling at the gallows for their raw material. The cadaver gave them purpose, whether it was to confirm what was explicated in a classic textbook, to find a new structure, or to pass on the accumulated anatomical knowledge to a succeeding generation.

At the same time that the fallacies propagated by Galen's animal dissections continued to be disproven, and major discoveries about the body's internal structures were being made by William Harvey and others, anatomists educated classes of would-be surgeons and physicians. Leading a class in the study of the body's morphology meant revealing layer by layer the systems and organs that make up the meaty human interior. Adding a sculptor's eye like that of Fredrick Ruysch, and anatomy — like the paintings in which it is depicted — was raised to a form of art ... a three-dimensional figure or a performance piece. To dissect is to demonstrate, which an anatomist does by wielding a scalpel on stage or behind the scenes. When public dissection was part of a capital sentence, anatomists skinned the bodies of criminals to bind books. When the great medical collections were being assembled, cadavers of average and anomalous men and women were stripped to salvage their skeletons. Anatomists embalmed cadavers wholesale, suspending them or standing them up in their private and institutional collections. Sometimes they hid them in their homes, keeping their cleaned or cured parts a secret until it was safe to reveal their majestic specimens. Sometimes they gathered their colleagues around them to bear witness to the moment the specimen was snipped.

The dissectors of earlier times and today have had the ability to mold bodies into anatomical marvels curated for future generations in medical museums, or to hold an audience spellbound by cutting cadavers apart. What these bodies symbolized for the anatomists and those who saw their work — during their lifetimes or long afterward — had much to do with the age in which they lived. During the Renaissance, Europeans crowded into newly-built anatomy theaters to see for themselves how the hand of God manifested itself in the internal workings of the human body. The revolutionary anatomist Andreas Vesalius was teaching those who watched in such an engrossing way that knowledge of anatomy came firsthand, not at arm's length through the published mistakes of predecessors. As the history of anatomy unfolded in the eighteenth and early nineteenth centuries, throngs of commoners clamored after an execution to ensure that the sentence to be hanged and publicly dissected was carried out to its ignominious end. The lesson to the audience, as depicted in William Hogarth's famous illustration, was that crime does not pay. The moral took the form of the undraped corpse picked apart in front of friends and neighbors — and perhaps skinned to make manifest the metaphorical book of the body. For Victorians watching the much-anticipated unwrapping and examination of an Egyptian mummy, Thomas Pettigrew was dissecting another culture for his well-heeled audience, not merely pulling apart an ancient and exotic human corpse. But early in the twentieth century, public dissection went underground. The cadaver came to signify privileged knowledge as witnessing and participating in dissection became the prerogative of doctors and doctors-to-be as part of their professional development. To revisit how the doors of the anatomy theater were opened to the public, closed to those without credentials, and then thrown open again, let us take a seat as the anatomist takes the stage...

"But it is, perhaps, this very impossibility of gazing within our bodies which makes the sight of the interior of other bodies so compelling." — Jonathan Sawday, *The Body Emblazoned: Dissection and the Human Body in Renaissance Culture* (1995)

Definitions of Dissection and Autopsy

Before we make the first incision, let's clarify the difference between a dissection and an autopsy, since the words are sometimes used interchangeably. Both words have Latin roots, both came into usage in English in the seventeenth century, and both mean to open up a dead body, but to autopsy a corpse is to *inspect* its internal structure and to dissect it is to *display* its internal structure. An autopsy, also known as a postmortem examination ("post" for short), is conducted to determine the cause of death, and may be medical or forensic in nature. A dissection is performed — often before an audience, as the definition suggests — to demonstrate human anatomy, either in part or in whole. In many historical accounts, an "anatomy" is not only the interior structure of the human body, but a synonym for the dissection of that body. Therefore, to put the pairing in verb form, a corpse may be *autopsied* to see how a person died, or *anatomized* to show how he or she lived.

In addition to a confusing terminology, the postmortem opening of the body for medico-legal reasons and for educational motivations share an overlapping history. According to scholar Andrea Carlino (1999), it was autopsy that seems to have paved the way for anatomical dissection. Forensic examination of the body's interior was done several decades before anatomies were carried out in Bologna and Venice, and autopsy in Paris preceded anatomical dissection by more than seventy years. On the other hand, historian Katherine Clarke points out that dissections were done in Italy as early as 1286 and were sometimes warranted to assess sainthood (van Dijck 2005), while recorded autopsies — says researcher Roger French (1999) — date to 1302, when surgeon Bartolomeo Varignana was ordered by a judge to open the body of Azzolino degli

Onesti, and confirmed that the man had not been poisoned. To further obfuscate the issue, consider similar events in Rome and Paris. The hospital autopsies to determine cause of death that Italian anatomist Bartolomeo Eustachi conducted in the sixteenth century established a theater of sorts that the public was allowed to attend, thus becoming true lessons in anatomy (Carlino 1999). The public dissections that French anatomist Jean Riolan the younger carried out in the anatomy theater in the seventeenth century were correlated to pathology, which made dissection forensic and disease something to be observed in a dissected body (French 1999).

The lack of clarification continued in the following centuries and has not ended in our own time. When ancient Egyptian mummies were unwrapped in the nineteenth and early twentieth centuries, the events were reported alternately as dissections or as autopsies. The public or semi-private search was for amulets more than evidence of disease, but preference for the term "autopsy" seems to be dictated by the dissector's affiliation with a professional institution. "Autopsies" were not done by amateurs in their drawing rooms. Nineteenth-century American showman P.T. Barnum used the word "autopsy" in the advertising copy for a procedure which did have the stated purpose of determining the age of the deceased. This

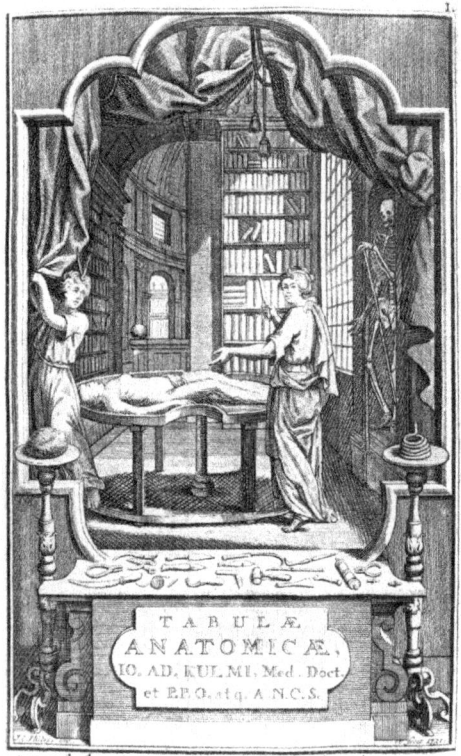

The title page of a 1755 edition of his anatomical text shows German anatomist Johann Adam Kulmus beginning a dissection, with his instruments lying on a table in the foreground (*Wellcome Images*).

Definitions of Dissection and Autopsy

postmortem was carried out by a doctor, but I have included the examination in this book because of the way it compares to the events performed in anatomy theaters for the primary purpose of entertaining the public. This book concludes with the entertainment offered by contemporary German anatomist Gunther von Hagens, who deliberately chooses to characterize the public dissection he performed as an "autopsy," perhaps to skirt the language of Britain's Anatomy Act and despite the fact that the cause of death in this case was already known. My rationale for including autopsies in this book on public dissection is when their public nature overrides any medical or legal concerns, and when the observed act of opening of the body supersedes what—besides the organs and structures—is found within.

Dissection Chronology

Third Century B.C.E.

Anatomy became a recognized discipline in Alexandria, and Herophilus — universally acknowledged as the "father of anatomy" — is believed to have been the first person to perform a public dissection. He systematized the anatomical description of the human body, and performed some 600 dissections during his career.

Second Century C.E.

Anatomical theory was disseminated by Galen, who dissected animals and extrapolated what he found to human dissection. His misapplied teachings dominated for some 1,500 years, during which time the practice of human dissection was kept alive by Arab physicians.

Thirteenth Century

The Roman Catholic Church prohibited the mutilation of human bodies in an attempt to curb the practice of reducing the remains of Christian crusaders to bones so they could be brought home as relics.

Fourteenth Century

With the sanction of the Pope, Mondino de Liuzzi completely anatomized two human bodies in 1315 — the first post–Alexandrian human dissection. For the next few centuries, dissection was carried out in a religious context, as a demonstration of God's design and a moral lesson about the brevity of life.

Fifteenth Century

By the end of the century, educational dissection was being carried out at the main universities of Europe, including Vienna, Prague, and Tubingen. The dissections followed a standard format in which the professor read from a medical text, a dissector exposed the structure being discussed, and an ostensor pointed to it. Dissections were held outdoors, in makeshift rooms, or in temporary structures. Anatomists began to take measures to ensure the anonymity of the cadaver. Artists including Michelangelo and Leonardo da Vinci observed or conducted their own dissections to more accurately portray the human figure. Dissection scenes, like those painted by Rembrandt, became a genre in Holland. The first permanent anatomical theater was erected in Padua in 1497.

Sixteenth Century

The first documented dissection in Rome took place in 1512.

A small number of bodies of executed criminals were allotted to barber-surgeons for dissection by James IV of Scotland in 1506 and Henry VIII of England in 1540. Attendance at public dissections increased. In the second half of the century, Vesalius initiated a seismic shift in the study of anatomy when he refuted the prevailing theories of Galen, recommending and practicing direct observation from the dissected human cadaver. Permanent anatomical theaters were erected in Leiden and Bologna.

Seventeenth Century

Permanent anatomical theaters were built in several European cities, including Copenhagen, Uppsala, Amsterdam, and Paris. Public dissections adhered to formal seating arrangements by seniority, but laws had to be enacted to control unruly crowds. Bodysnatching began — and continued well into (and in the U.S., beyond) the nineteenth century — to fill the demand for subjects to dissect that was not met by legal allotments from the gallows or poorhouse.

Eighteenth Century

The First Anatomy Act was passed in England in 1752 and gave judges the latitude to substitute dissection for gibbeting in sentencing the worst crimes. In 1783, executions were no longer public, and the gallows in London were moved inside Newgate Prison, after which the bodies to be dissected were transferred to the adjacent Surgeon's Hall. The Guild of Barber-Surgeons became a more professional organization, moving into the Royal College. Now that nearly every medical school had its own anatomical theater, academics began to question the intended educational purpose of the public dissection.

Nineteenth Century

Infamous bodysnatchers William Burke and William Hare were brought to trial, and Burke was executed and dissected. Bodysnatching flourished and frequently provoked riots when discovered, although authorities often turned a blind eye. In 1832, the Second Anatomy Act was passed in England, abolishing the penalty of dissection for murder. Instead, it authorized the release of unclaimed bodies to anatomists, which shifted the pool of available cadavers from executed felons to the poor. By the end of the American Civil War, most of the United States had passed anatomy laws sanctioning the dissection of executed prisoners and the bodies of the unclaimed dead. By mid-century, dissection had become an essential part of the medical curriculum, but *public* dissection was seen as crude and an embarrassment to the field. It was fashionable in England and America to attend private "unrollings" or public lectures in which ancient Egyptian mummies were dissected.

Twentieth Century

Photographs of students in their smocks gathered around the cadaver they are dissecting became a rite of passage in American medical schools. After World War II, whole-body donations accounted for more than 70 percent of all dissections. The public no longer had access to the dissection of cadavers, which occurred out of sight in medical institutions.

Twenty-First Century

Gross anatomy, which includes dissection of a human cadaver, is still a required course for first-year medical students. At the same time, its necessity is sometimes questioned as the technology improves for conducting "virtual dissections" electronically. German anatomist Gunther von Hagens stirs controversy by performing a dissection before a live British audience which was later broadcast on television.

Introduction

Cadavers function like books: as their metaphorical leaves are turned, knowledge is gained. Dissectors have always thought so, and have found many ways of expressing this. When London anatomist and surgeon John Hunter was meeting with the father of a potential student in 1789, he was asked which textbooks would be studied. "Hunter simply led the way to the dissecting room, where several open cadavers lay, and declared, 'These are the books your son will learn under my direction, the others are fit for very little'" (Moore 2005). Hunter's contemporary Jean-Joseph Sue the Elder wrote, "In the process of dissecting, our searches through the entrails of Nature herself, who becomes a book for us, & the impressions which stay with us are infinitely more sensible than those acquired by other studies" (Simon 2002). Guaranteeing direct dissecting experience to complement lectures and demonstrations gave private anatomy professors a selling point when offering their courses to would-be surgeons.

By the eighteenth century, the discipline of anatomy had progressed beyond books by Galen and others who extrapolated the physiology of humans based on the dissection of animals (known as "zootomy," a term used since the seventeenth century to distinguish it from "androtomy" or "anthropotomy," the dissection of man). Andreas Vesalius had made his mark two hundred years earlier and left the anatomists who followed a textbook based on the actual dissection of human cadavers. But his seven-volume *De humani corporis fabrica [On the fabric of the human body]* not only mapped out the human interior with authority, it encouraged all other anatomists to look within the corpse, to learn from direct observation rather than second-hand, to break free of the constraints that kept the lofty physician elevated above the dissecting table and the lowly

Introduction

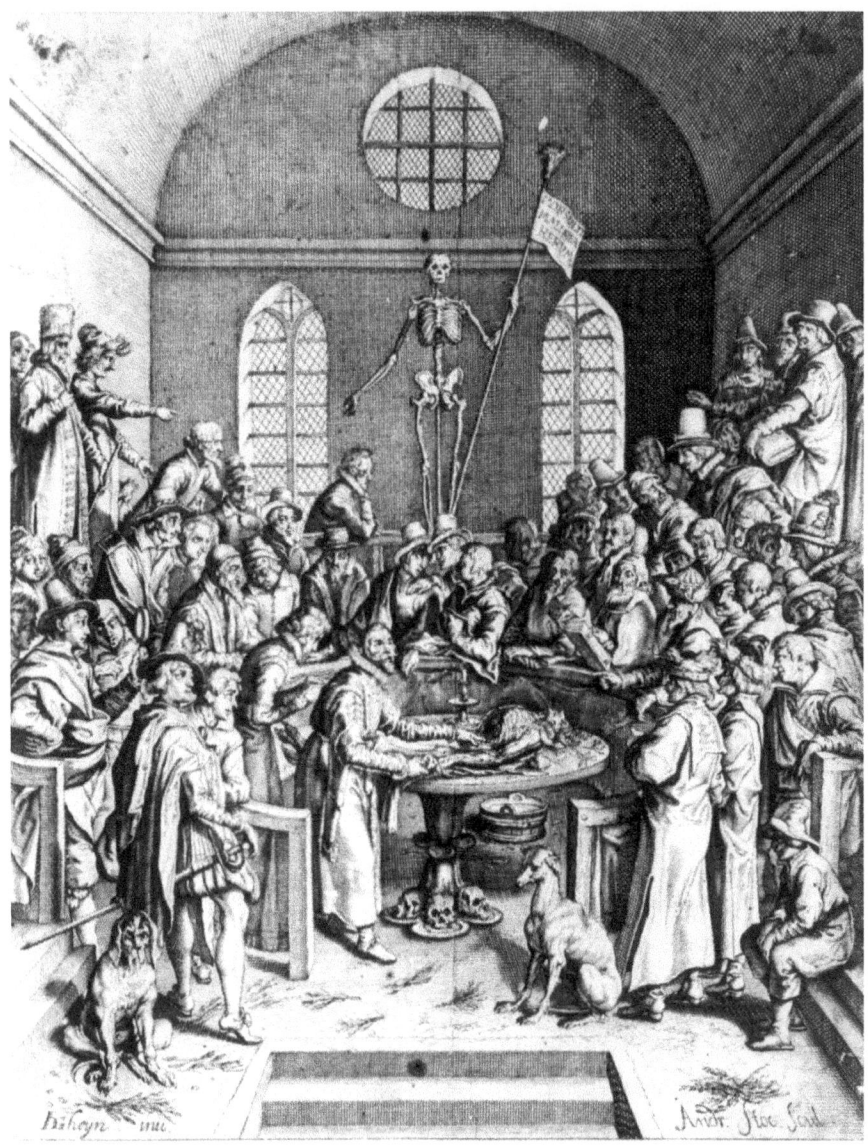

This print from 1616 depicts medical students observing an anatomical dissection. A skeleton stands to the rear and skulls surround the table's pedestal. Two dogs are seated in the foreground and a bucket sits behind the table, all of which are presumably ready to accept the scraps (*courtesy National Library of Medicine*).

and uneducated dissector doing the dirty work. Vesalius urged those who lectured about anatomy to do the cutting themselves. He convinced others by his example that the human body was a more important body of knowledge than the mistake-prone tome they were reciting from their pulpits.

In the pre–Renaissance dissecting theater, the professor recited from a medical text while the assistant opened the cadaver and tried to illustrate the spoken word with swipes of his scalpel. Even when the text diverged from the body before them, that misinformed though accepted text was understood to be correct. The seemingly anomalous corpse was the *recipient* of the authorial word, and was made to exemplify it. In the subsequent dissecting theater of Andreas Vesalius, the professor took his place next to the cadaver and became both lecturer and dissector. He read from the text, but more importantly he was able to revise that textual authority as the dissection disagreed with it. "The opened body has replaced the opened book as the source of anatomical knowledge, suggesting that responsibility for knowledge now lies within its exposed interiority," writes Maria Angel (2004). She goes on to explain that as the canonical text disappeared into the flesh, the word was made thing. What was *read* and what was *seen* merged, mapping representation back onto being.

For Vesalius, the body was not only a book, it was a primary source. Others felt the same way. Quattrocento and cinquecento artists including Leonardo da Vinci and Michelangelo took great pains — and great risks — to privately dissect the musculature beneath the skin of the dead so they could accurately portray its appearance as it rippled beneath the skin of their living models. Anatomist John Bell was such a gifted artist that he insisted on illustrating his own dissection manuals so that the books would match the bodies faithfully (some would say *too* faithfully), without aesthetics getting in the way. From its tentative beginnings in the Middle Ages, dissection was taken up in the Renaissance as a religious celebration. The dissection was public — sanctioned and sanctified. The body was a book, but it could be characterized as a devotional. Its pages were read by candlelight, the attention given to it was ceremonial, and its inner workings revealed the hand of God. The anatomical illustrations of the time depict cadavers participating in their own dissections, with skeletons and musclemen acting out the ancient Greek adage "Know thyself." The body was, in this sense, an autobiography.

In *Culture and the Human Body*, anthropologist John W. Burton (2001) writes, "The human body can be likened to a cultural mirror." With this quote — derivative of "The social body constrains the way the physical body is perceived" by Mary Douglas (1996) — Burton suggests that our bodies are reflections of the societies in which we live. What was for the medieval dissector an interior that remained dark and for the most part unexplored had become, for the Renaissance anatomist, a challenge, an obligation to shed light on the internal workings that we all share. Burton reasons that since the body is an image of society, our bodies are not entirely our own: "The fact is that while we regard our bodies as the fundamental basis of our intimate identity and sense of self, the body is a public medium and a public possession" (Burton 2001). This is meant to be understood in the abstract, and holds true in life and in death. But it also has a less symbolic application to the cadaver on the dissecting table: "We are not really social beings until we are 'read' or interpreted by some other person. Our physical and psychic being is dependent upon some kind of audience" (Burton 2001). Just as living persons require being "read" by others to acquire their social selves, dead bodies must be deciphered to form an understanding of our collective physical self.

Dissecting cadavers publicly, especially in a punitive context, made an open book of the body. The secrets inside our physical selves were shared with the masses in an often unruly event. Students of the university turned out for a lesson, but on the other side of the anatomy theater members of the community with no medical qualifications came to gawk. They were drawn to the nineteenth-century spectacle of a human corpse being dismantled. They were eager to see the second half of the legal sentence to be "hanged and publicly dissected" carried out. And if the executed felon happened to be female, they were thrilled at the opportunity to witness retributive justice and at the same time to have an excuse to stare at the unveiled female form, as gory as it may be under those circumstances. But it was not just the medically uninitiated for whom the body was a book of erotica. Renowned French scientist Georges Cuvier was tickled to be able to open that book in the form of the newly deceased "Hottentot Venus." He invited his colleagues to observe the dissection of this anthropological specimen whose storied sex organs had remained a mystery while she was alive and only exhibited herself clothed. The men gathered around her corpse with their notebooks and sketch pads and watched Cuvier not only reveal her elongated labia, but excise and preserve them.

With this mindset among professionals as well as the general public, it was not too much of a stretch to make the book-body metaphor manifest by harvesting the skin of a cadaver and using it to enclose the pages of an appropriate written work. Men of earlier centuries were known to have bound novels by the Marquis de Sade in women's skin and to have sandwiched pornographic novels between covers wrapped with the skin of female breasts. But only a small subset of those who practiced this particularly literal incarnation of the merging of book and body were fetishists. Anthropodermic books, as they are known, have been bound since the fourteenth century, and several examples still exist in libraries, museums, and private collections. Researcher Holbrook Jackson acknowledges that the production and collection of such books is decidedly morbid, but writes:

> Having thus established that human hides have been tanned, and that the hides are usable, it requires no ingenuity to extend its use to other purposes and, having regard, as the lawyers say, to the close relationship between books and men, their humane behavior, etc., I find the application of this sort of leather to books a logical if macabre enterprise [Jackson 1932].

There were specialized human-leather bindings to serve anthropologists (*Das Rätsel des Menschen [The Riddle of Mankind]* in 1910), spiritualists (a book bound in the skin of the "Witch of Yorkshire" in the late nineteenth century), and the devout (a Book of Hours in 1671 and a Qur'an in 1867). There were anthropodermic bindings that had been sparked by the French Revolution (*Constitution de la Republique Français,* Jean-Jacques Rousseau's *Social Contract,* and Thomas Paine's *The Rights of Man*) and anthropological works about race bound in African American skin. Some anthropodermic books were self-designated by the owners of the skin that was then tanned postmortem. But what is of interest here are two categories of anthropodermic bindings: medical treatises bound in the skin of cadavers and trial transcripts bound in the skin of condemned prisoners who became cadavers as soon as they were executed...

There was a pocket of doctors trained or practicing in Philadelphia in the 1800s who rebound certain books in their libraries (Andreas Vesalius' 1568 *De Humani Corporis Fabrica* and Hans Holbein's 1816 *Dance of Death* were favorites) in human leather. One of them was physician Dr. John Stockton Hough, who rebound three gynecology texts in women's skin. These included Robert Couper's *Speculations on the Mode and Appearances of Impregnation in the Human Female* (1789) and Carolus Drelincurtius's *De Conceptione Adversaria* (1686). The skin used to bind the books, which are now owned by the College of Physicians of Philadelphia, was said to have come from either the twenty-eight-year-old Irish-American widow in whom Dr. Hough had diagnosed the city's first case of trichinosis or a patient who had died of consumption in the hospital. Of course, Pennsylvania was by no means the only place where this was carried out. A collection of gynecological essays originally published in 1663 was bound in Paris for Dr. Ludovic Bouland at the turn of the twentieth century. Bouland had obtained the skin from the body of a woman, presumably unclaimed, who died in the hospital when he was a medical student.

As Mirjam Foot (1993), a leading scholar of bookbinding history, reveals, many books printed in the seventeenth and eighteenth centuries were purchased in sheets, to be bound as the owner wished. Only when this was done in a way that would reflect the literary content within would it preserve a direct relationship between a book and its binding that has since become standard. The nineteenth-century anatomists were influenced by a number of convergences at the time. Collecting had become fashionable, taxidermic preservation techniques had been developed, an interest in curiosities had been provoked by American showman P.T. Barnum and others, and individual medical museums and libraries were becoming institutionalized upon their owners' deaths. But perhaps the factor that was most responsible for this odd fad was recent legislation. Anatomy legislation in America and abroad made obtaining cadavers for dissection easier, which made their skin a ready material for doctors. Some of these bodies came straight from the gallows, and anatomists were legally obliged to publicly dissect them, so using their tanned skin to bind their court documents must have seemed only appropriate. Such was the fate of James Johnson (1818), George Cudmore (1830), and the three executed men discussed below.

William Corder ran a 300-acre farm in Polstead, Suffolk, England, with his mother when he took up with a twenty-four-year-old woman by the name of Maria Marten in 1826. Corder was known as a ladies' man and Marten had many admirers. She already had a young son, Thomas Henry, by one of them. She and Corder rendezvoused on his land in a red barn and the following year she gave birth to his child. She had hoped this would lead to a marriage proposal, but the month-old child sickened and died. Corder did ask for her hand in marriage, but insisted that she dress in male attire — so as not to attract notice — and meet him in the red barn for the journey to Ipswich. He returned from Ipswich without her, explaining that she had remained behind. He again left and wrote to her father that they were living on the Isle of Wight. He provided continued excuses for Maria's failure to contact her family or send for her son. After having a dream that Maria was dead and buried in the red barn, her stepmother convinced Maria's father to investigate. With a friend, he excavated a soft spot in the barn floor and uncovered a mangled, decomposed body in a bag. The corpse was dressed in men's clothing and was clearly that of his daughter.

The police tracked Corder down in Brentford. He had taken a wife and they were running a boarding house. He was returned to Polstead for an inquest and confessed that he had accidentally shot Maria with a pistol after they had argued about their deceased child. On August 11, 1828, three days after the trial had ended, William Corder was hanged for the sensational "murder in the red barn." Thousands turned out to witness the execution, and heard Corder confess a second time on the scaffold. After a final prayer, the rope supporting the platform was severed and his body dropped. The hangman grabbed him around the waist to finish his suffering, during which Corder raised his hands several times. But his agony was over in a matter of minutes and his body went limp. The body was taken down an hour later, removed to Shire Hall, and cut open from throat to abdomen to expose the muscles. Then, clothed only in trousers and stockings, it was exposed to the public until 6 o'clock that evening. At that time, the head and face were shaven in preparation for molds to be made: a bust by Mr. Child of Suffolk and a death mask by Mr. Mazzotti of Cambridge. Journalist James Curtis remarks, "The countenance did not appear much changed, except that the under lip was drawn down so as to expose the teeth in the upper jaw: this had the effect, in a great degree, of obliterating the indentation which in life was very observable on the top of the chin. There appeared to be a considerable effusion of blood about the neck and throat, occasioned by the pressure of the rope in the moment of strangulation." The hangman claimed Corder's clothing as his right, and the body was removed to the county hospital.

The dissection of William Corder's body was conducted over two days by Dr. George Creed and his colleague Dr. Smith at the West Suffolk Hospital. Several other medical men were in attendance, drawn from both nearby and considerable distances, including a Dr. Yellowby from Norwich hospital who wanted to observe the mucous membranes. Dr. Creed reported that the following organs and structures were dissected on the first day and described to those present: the sternum; the lungs, which had adhesions due to pleuritic disease and were gorged with blood; the heart, filled with a small amount of serum and a large amount of fluid blood consistent with sudden death; the trachea and stomach, both found to be inflamed; the large and small intestines; the kidneys, which were somewhat enlarged; and the bladder, which was contracted, likely due to the shock to the nervous system. Creed reports, "An interesting discussion took place, respecting the cause of death from hanging — whether it was suffocation or pressure upon the spinal cord. From the circumstance of the chest and shoulders of Corder being observed to heave several minutes after the drop fell, it was generally admitted that death most probably took place from the latter cause." The brain was not examined, to maintain the integrity of the skull for the skeleton. The head was cast by a Mr. Childs and a phrenological examination was made showing the parts indicating intellectual qualities to be lacking in proportion.

The second day allowed for minute dissection of the heart, and the dissection and casting of the muscles of the arm. In addition, the results of the phrenological examination revealed that Corder had the following traits: secretiveness, acquisitiveness, destructiveness, philoprogenitiveness (love of offspring), and imitativeness. Additional details supplied by a Mr. J. Macintyre dismissed phrenology as a presumptuous pseudoscience, but added for the record that Corder's organ of intellectual development was small, as were the areas signifying benevolence and veneration, but those of combativeness, adhesiveness, cautiousness, and firmness were pronounced. A cast of the cranium was sent to Johann Gaspar Spurzheim (1776–1832), one of the initial proponents of phrenology, for his opinion, which he duly offered, concluding that "the natural moral character of such a head is formed by animal feelings, deprived of self-esteem, firmness, conscientiousness, and reflection, and very little assisted by benevolence, veneration, and ideality — his internal monitor, therefore, is quite wanting." Corder's body measured five feet six inches and was noted to be muscular and well-proportioned. "The body was perfectly healthy, and every organ sound," writes Mr. Macintyre, dismissing any disease of the lungs and drawing more attention to the inflammation in the stomach and intestines, which exhibited throughout "a fine vermilion blush," and the corrugation of the stomach which, had the cause of death not been known, may have suggested arsenic poisoning. Lastly, marks on the neck were scars (possibly syphilitic, and not tuberculous) or marks made by the hanging itself. Remnants of the dissection of the infamous "Red Barn Murderer" are on display at Moyse's Hall Museum in Bury St. Edmunds. These include one of many casts made of the original death mask in the Norwich Castle Museum; the death bust, which was examined by phrenologists; the scalp, which was preserved with a single ear attached; and Dr. Creed's copy of the account of the crime and trial — *The Mysterious Murder of Maria Marten* by James Curtis — which he had bound in 1828 from skin that he had removed from Corder's back.

John Horwood grew up in the village of Hanham Mills near Bristol, England. At the age of seventeen, his relationship with local girl Eliza Balsom soured and he began to stalk and threaten her. When he saw her walking along the brook with a new boyfriend, he took out his frustrations by hurling a stone at her. Unfortunately for them both, that stone hit her eye. The wound — or by other accounts, the hole drilled to relieve the pressure — became infected, and Eliza died a few weeks later. Horwood resisted arrest, but was taken into custody. He was sentenced to

Introduction

be hanged and publicly dissected. The first half of the sentence was carried out on April 13, 1821, above the gatehouse door of Bristol's newly built gaol. A large crowd gathered for the event, jostling so as not to fall into the New Cut River and purchasing commemorative handbills. Horwood's family had hoped to spirit his body away via the river, but were thwarted by the gaol authorities who delivered it to the Bristol Royal Infirmary.

The second half of Horwood's sentence was performed by surgeon Richard Smith, who dissected the body before a crowd of eighty of his students. But Dr. Smith did more than just carry out the letter of the law. He harvested, articulated, and curated the skeleton, which he housed in a wooden cabinet and showed to his houseguests. He also skinned the body, and paid to have the skin tanned and used to bind a book of all the papers relating to John Horwood's case, including the detailed notes he had made during the dissection. The hand-tooled book was shelved in the infirmary's library for decades until it was transferred to its present location at the Bristol Record Office. The University of Bristol recently agreed to cremate the skeleton and release the ashes to Mary Halliwell of Greater Manchester, who has traced her ancestry to Horwood. She hopes to honor his parents' wishes by burying his remains — including the anthropodermic book — in the churchyard where his family is interred. With the help of a local funeral director, the Halliwell family planned the burial of what was left of John Horwood to coincide to the hour with the 190th anniversary of the execution of his body.

Twelve years later and an ocean away in 1833, thirty-one-year-old French immigrant Antoine LeBlanc took up residence in the basement of the Sayres residence in Morristown, New Jersey. He had been offered room and board in exchange for feeding the hogs and chopping the wood. He became disenchanted with the arrangement in less than three weeks and bludgeoned Judge Samuel Sayres, his wife Sarah, and their servant Phoebe to death, escaping with valuables from the house. After LeBlanc was tracked down, he was tried and a verdict rendered by the jury in twenty minutes. Judge Gabriel Ford sentenced him to be hanged by the neck until dead, and then delivered to surgeon Dr. Isaac Canfield for dissection. His execution on the village green was attended by a crowd upwards of 10,000, most of them from out of town.

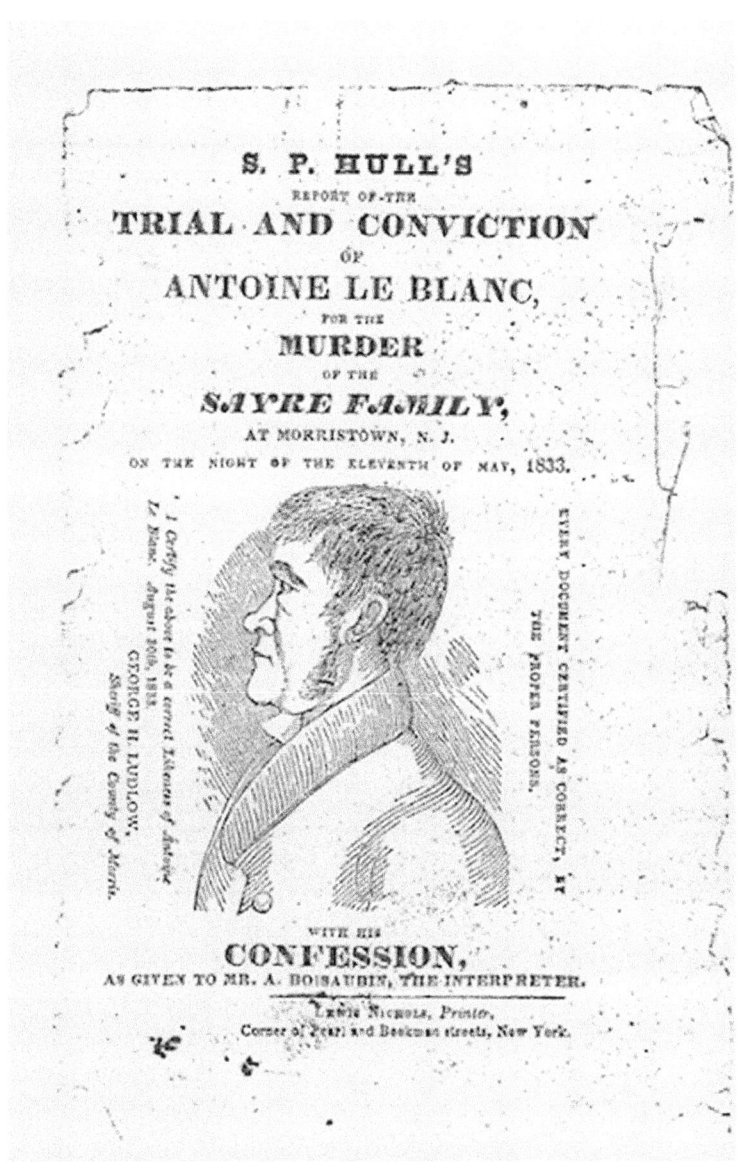

The cover of an account by S.P. Hull of the 1833 murders of the Sayre Family of New Jersey that resulted in Antoine LeBlanc's execution and dissection. A jury found LeBlanc guilty in twenty minutes. He was hanged on the village green and conveyed across the street to the surgeon's office for dissection. His skeleton was never articulated, but his bones turned up decades later in the county clerk's office. Some of the souvenirs made from his skin are still in private hands (*courtesy WeirdNJ.com*).

INTRODUCTION

After LeBlanc was put to death, his body was conveyed across the street to the surgeon's office, where it was the subject of electrical experiments by Dr. Canfield and Dr. Isaac Henry. The doctors cast LeBlanc's face in plaster, then removed his skin and had it delivered to the nearby Atno Tannery. There it was tanned and crafted into keepsakes: wallets, purses, lampshades, and book jackets. In addition, small strips of skin — each authenticated with the signature of Sheriff George Ludlow — were sold on the streets. Decades later, rumors that Dr. Canfield had preserved and kept LeBlanc's skeleton were dispelled when renovations of the county clerk's office revealed the unarticulated bones in a box in 1893. The death mask and a change purse were found among the possessions of Carl Scherzer, an unofficial town historian, upon his death in 1995, and others of the gruesome souvenirs are believed to remain in private collections.

How the raw pieces of a dissected body can be transformed into medical and legal book-bindings, and even curios sought after by the general public, is explained by French theorist Julia Kristeva. With her "abjection theory," she sheds light on how we view anthropodermic bindings and other items made by harvesting the skin of the corpse. Kristeva defines the abject as those things that disturb order and identity, for which we have both a repulsion and a fascination. The abject threatens to destroy life, and is therefore expelled, but also helps to define it. The corpse is the ultimate in abjection and — as one of the most basic forms of pollution — is usually excluded by ritual. In the case of human leather, tanning has removed the possibility of decay, forestalling its expulsion. In addition, it has been crafted into an object, and Kristeva explains that art is one way of purifying the abject. Another way that many anthropodermic books have avoided abjection is by remaining within the realm of science and religion. "The corpse, seen without God and outside of science, is the utmost of abjection. It is death infecting life" (Kristeva 1982). For the medical men of the nineteenth century, binding a renowned anatomy text in the skin of its subject — the human body — was a tribute to science, and to God who was responsible for our bodies and our knowledge of them.

The scholarly tradition in which text is seen as both dead and alive also gives reason to the binding of books in human skin, since human

Introduction

leather, too, is both dead and retains a presence. Those who practiced anthropodermic bookbinding merged the book and the body in such a way that the resulting objects allow identity to outlast the body. Even if that identity is infamous, when the book contains the life of a person — anthropodermic on the outside, biographical on the inside — immortality in the physical sense is almost certain. When William Corder was hanged for the notorious 1827 shooting death of his lover described in the newspapers as "The Murder in the Red Barn," the skin of his back was removed after his subsequent dissection and was used by the anatomist to bind James Curtis' The Mysterious Murder of Maria Marten — thereby assuring that Corder's name lives on to this day and his story is retold to the visitors of the Edinburgh museum where the anthropodermic book is on display. But coupled with this secular immortality is the idea of redemption, with the book serving as a reminder that Corder paid for his crime with his life *and his hide.*

In his classic *The Hour of Our Death*, Philippe Ariès catalogs the connections between books and immortality. Ariès notes several themes in the Holy Bible, such as the appearance of the names of believers in God's book (Daniel 12:1), that will be opened at the end of the world (Revelations 5:1). A corresponding *liber vitae* (book of lives) contained the names of benefactors of the Church that were read during prayer services. By the thirteenth century, the *liber vitae* was no longer a census of the faithful, but a weighing of the thoughts, words, and deeds of the individual: "Life is a body of facts that can be itemized and summarized in a book," Ariès (1982) writes. The book is a biography, but also an account book of good versus evil, so that by the next century it had become not a book of the elect, but a book of the damned. The anthropodermic books of Corder's crime and Horwood's trial and dissection perpetuate their guilt in the physical world. If these men had donated their bodies to medical science, instead of being subject to compulsory legal dissection, they may have been understood to have expiated their sins to a degree.

For those few eighteenth- and nineteenth-century individuals like forward-thinking philosopher Jeremy Bentham, who bequeathed their remains for anatomical education, the body was — theoretically speaking — a library book. After it transitioned from subject to object, it could transmit knowledge if shared. The same could be said of prepaid volunteers like bodysnatcher "Old Cunny," even though their motives for accepting money during life for the right to dissect their bodies after death were less altruistic than avaricious. The families of African American slaves who were unfortunate enough to require hospitalization at the end of their lives found that they were unable to lay their loved ones to rest. To their owners and the medical institution, their bodies were nothing more than an account book in which the use of their corpse balanced the cost of their care. But even those who escaped this fate and were buried had a good chance of ending up on the dissecting table, since bodysnatchers preyed on the occupants of African American burial grounds. Nobody—*no body*—was safe, however, as anatomist Sir Astley Cooper made clear to British Parliament when he boasted that he could get his hands on any corpse if he so desired.

In his paper "Bodies of Thought" (1991) and his book *Flesh in the Age of Reason* (2003), Roy Porter notes that during the Enlightenment of the eighteenth century, philosophers reasoned that in the early history of the human race, people analogized everything in terms of the workings of the human body, thus the body was "good to think with" (1991). For the anatomists of that time, the body was good to *build with*. For master embalmers Honoré Fragonard and Frederik Ruysch, bodies were components of a scrapbook of sorts. Their respective anatomical cabinets were chronologies of their projects that isolated and highlighted the body's systems, in the case of Fragonard's myologies and angiologies, and disguised the body's detritus as landscape, in the tableaux of Ruysch. Modeler Clemente Susini preferred to translate the book of the body into wax, remaking it as a three-dimensional figure that rivaled that maintained its integrity without being embalmed and offered the volume that textbook illustrations lacked. By the nineteenth century, Cooper and his fellow anatomists found the body indispensable to *teach with*. Whether they were on the faculty of a university or tutoring private pupils, these dissectors had to avail themselves of the services of the bodysnatchers to meet their need for the hands-on textbooks and manuals that were the human body. To the students of that time and later, cadavers were not only the books they studied, but rosters to which they metaphorically signed their names. Teams of doctors in training secured their educational credentials by sharing the dissection of a body and, beginning shortly after photography was invented, had themselves photographed with this most important resource.

Writing just a few years ago, medical student Christine Montross (2007) describes how the cadaver functions as a book in more than an abstract way. Dissectors quickly learn that opening a body and opening a book have *physical* similarities: "The skin of the chest pulls back easily after we have made the incisions, and the body opens like a book." Similarly, contemporary German anatomist Gunther von Hagens, impresario of the BodyWorlds exhibits, experiences the process of preparing and posing preserved human bodies for display:

> The body, then, comprises a set of folded surfaces that can be opened like a book, and the process of inscription or engraving retheorized in terms of a process similar to flaying — the description of the incision drawn on the body in this case can refer to a process of writing as unsheathing [Angel 2004].

Von Hagens peels and positions his plastinated bodies to tell a particular truth about anatomy. Much of this truth is "spoken" by the raw flesh he exposes to museum-goers, who may never have been in such proximity to a human heart that was not in a jar or musculature that did not need to be exhibited behind glass. But von Hagens does not let the corpus of knowledge tell its own story. Instead, he constructs his own readings of the flesh (Hallam et al. 1999). The flayed man holds his heart in his hand; the runner's muscles stream behind him as if by his forward momentum. Emulating the anatomists and medical illustrators who preceded him with many of his poses, like Fragonard's "Rider on a Horse," today's best-known anatomist reminds us that the body may be a book, but one that is ripe for revision. It is, for him, a script to be restaged.

It is the *staging* of the body that has changed, with circumstance and with the personality and style of the anatomist. Cadavers were opened in hidden and claustrophobic spaces when the activity had to be shielded from the law, the Church, and the public. The stage was centered in temporary open-air structures and later in permanent skylit amphitheaters after it was realized that dissection of the human body was a necessary prerequisite to a career in surgery — and before it was thought to restrict the public from what was not always a learning experience. And corpses were dismantled in private dissection rooms and institutionalized anatomy laboratories to which only tuition-paying students had access, while members of the public were invited to attend ticketed cultural and educational performances in rented lecture halls. In one century, artists attended anatomy demonstrations side-by-side with doctors in training, so that they could accurately portray human musculature in their paintings. In a later century, a body would be pulled apart before an incited crowd that had just egged on the executioner at the subject's hanging. And more recently, as technology has allowed, exhibits of bodies in a permanent state of dissection have been staged in a scientific context and patronized by millions.

According to the *Oxford English Dictionary*, "to stage" is "to mount or put on (a spectacle)." Where human dissection is concerned, the parenthetical "spectacle" is in the eyes of the audience of the time — and in the minds of the scholars who followed. In many definitions of the word "spectacle," it is simply a public performance, a meaning which most all of the events described in this book fulfill. But the definition under which this particular history is predicated is one based on intent, the motivations of the anatomists of past and present. Within this volume, at least, "spectacle" has a slightly negative connotation. I define it as a public display or performance *intended to impress the audience with its scale or extravagance*. Under this definition, a public dissection that immediately followed a public execution was a spectacle, intended to posthumously shame the criminal, to continue to engage the already incited crowd, and to discourage future lawbreakers. An educational performance in an anatomy theater to which the public was invited was also a spectacle, offering compulsory participation of university faculty, a chance to see specially-seated dignitaries in addition to the dissection, and an opportunity to put the host city on the anatomical map. Demonstrations conducted within the halls of the university for the education of its students, or gatherings of paying pupils around the dissecting table in a professor's basement laboratory, were not spectacles — unless the dissectors meant them to be. Spectacles were created by anatomists, who performed their combination of art and science before a live audience or crafted specimens from the privately dissected cadaver that were presented en masse to the public in a museum. The anatomists' private cabinets became institutionalized the same way their human dissections eventually needed to be carried out within the halls of a university rather than in the open air or the home laboratory.

Whether a historical event was considered a spectacle at the time or deemed so by future eyes is a matter of degree. A villager in an earlier century watching a temporary anatomy theater being erected was impressed by the magnitude of the event to come, that it would merit such preparation, while to future eyes the structure may seem crude in comparison to later permanent theaters — and the rough and raucous dissection it would facilitate may seem cruder still. To a Victorian gentleman, a ticket to the unwrapping of a mummy by a notable scholar in a plush London venue was a prize, and an invitation a private unrolling by an amateur in his home was even more of a coup. The celebrity unrollers were invited to preside in the parlor or to pack the decorated auditorium, and purposed — as were the ancient mummies themselves — to awe the crowd, large or small. To the guest or patron of the time, the unwrapping was a delightful diversion. But to the modern mind, the sin was not in the spectacle, it was in the fact that both of these situations were less than scientific and robbed the future of linens, amulets, and often the mummies themselves that could have pushed forward Egyptology with reexamination and technological advancements. To us, the public dissection of one of P.T. Barnum's attractions to prove her great age was just the kind of spectacle for which the showman was known, and we can — with the benefit of hindsight — place it within his repertoire of fleecing a gullible public. To an excited ticket-holder at the time, however, it was a historic chance to see the world-renowned impresario officially proven or disproven in spectacular style.

What follows are groupings of anatomists and vignetted looks into their lives and times, from how they got their hands on the raw materials to what they did to those cadavers once in their clutches. The primary reason for dissecting the body was, of course, to see what was inside. After that was formally established and scientifically documented, the motivations were to demonstrate to others what had been learned about the corpse's contents to date, and to continue to revise and refine that knowledge by observing, experimenting, and using newly developed tools. In the course of their work, anatomists were called upon by the

INTRODUCTION

authorities to carry out their craft in front of others, not to necessarily to teach but to show. The dissection was an event, following a judicial hanging, scheduled to coincide with a civic festival, or arranged so that it could be attended by large numbers of paying patrons. While countless (and nameless) faculty anatomists have in fact taught tuition-paying students using the unsurpassed means of opening the body, the anatomists who took to the stage of the anatomy theater — or beckoned visitors to their fully-stocked anatomy cabinets — with the purpose of impressing their audience are the ones who are remembered.

1

Anatomists as Procurers of Cadavers

"The Reward of Cruelty" is one in a series of engravings by English artist William Hogarth in 1751. In the first image, a fictional subject named Tom Nero tortures a dog as a child, while his fellows brutalize other animals. In the second, he is shown in his adult occupation of hackney coach, now violently beating the horse that is no longer able to pull his carriage. In the third, Nero progresses to highway robbery and the cruel murder of the woman he has impregnated. And in the fourth and final scene, Tom's body has just been taken down from the gallows with the noose still around his neck. He is shown in an anatomical theater being dissected by surgeons before an audience of academics (wearing mortar-boards), clerics, physicians (wearing wigs), and gentlemen observers. The anatomists show as much care for him as he did for his victims. One participant puts out his eye, as Nero had done to his horse. As a group, they allow the dog beneath the table to devour his heart, as if taking revenge for the animal cruelty of his boyhood. The exaggerated expression on Nero's face is meant to heighten the viewers' horror and the skeleton being pointed to plainly illustrates his physical fate: he will fill a similar niche or cupboard, rather than being laid to rest in a grave. The verse beneath the print reads in part:

> Behold the Villain's dire disgrace!
> Not Death itself can end.
> He finds no peaceful Burial-Place,
> His breathless Corse, no friend...

Hogarth based the chief surgeon (seated in the high-backed chair) on the president of the Royal College of Surgeons, the setting on the Cutlerian theater near Newgate Prison, and the scene on the frontispiece to Vesalius' anatomy textbook (discussed below). The engravings were

DISSECTION ON DISPLAY

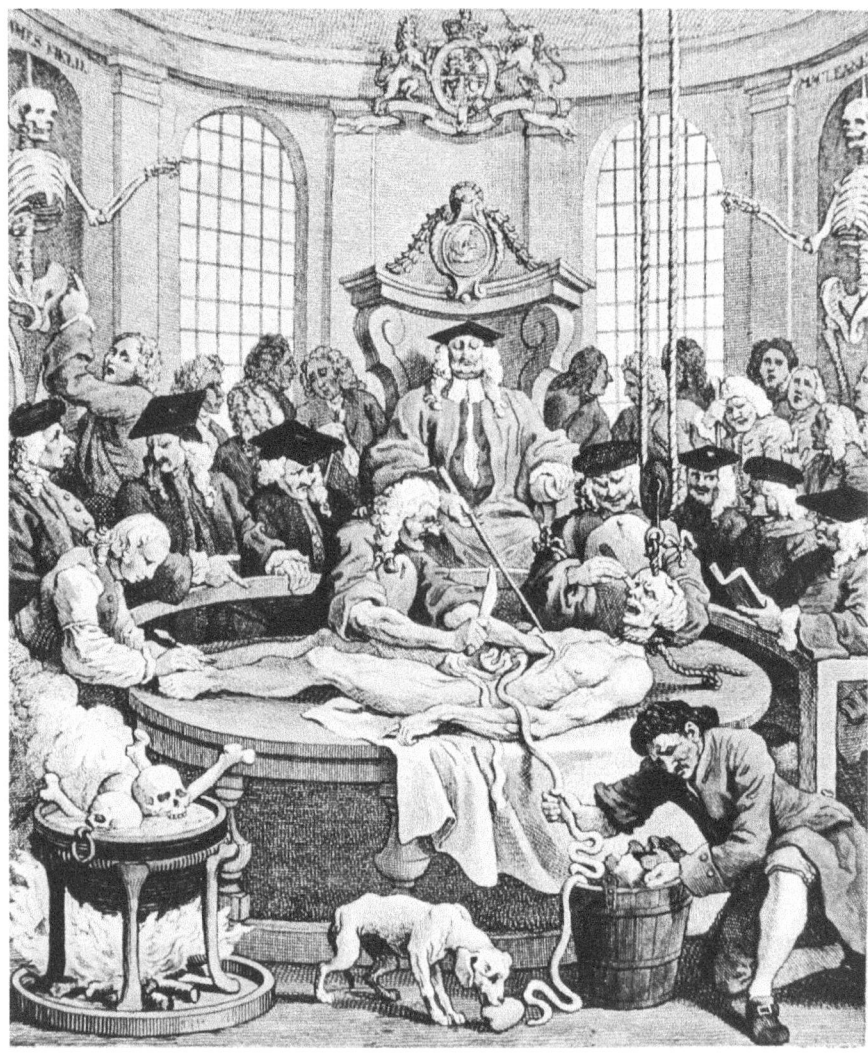

"The Four Stages of Cruelty: The Reward of Cruelty," the last in a series of 1751 engravings by William Hogarth intended to deromanticize the life of crime, after earlier illustrations document the stages of cruelty from an early age. Executed criminal Nero, who has been hanged at Tyburn, is being dissected in the Cutlerian anatomical theater near Newgate Prison. The chief surgeon is seated in the high-backed chair directing the dissector who cuts the body. The skeletons in the niches to right and left are remains of earlier dissected criminals, who were denied a Christian burial (*courtesy National Library of Medicine*).

printed cheaply with the intention that they would circulate among London's lower classes, which Hogarth — based on what he witnessed in the streets — felt were in need of moral instruction. They were also published in the *London Evening Post* along with commentary by an ordained minister about where the path of immoral behavior leads. Hogarth was pleased with the series, even though some of his contemporaries dismissed it as caricature, and history bore him out. By the early 1830s, cruelty to animals and the dissection of executed felons were outlawed.

In Britain, dissections were licensed in 1540 by Henry VIII through an act which specified that the Company of Barber-Surgeons "maie have and take without contridiction foure persons condempned adjudged and put to deathe for feloni ... for anatomies ... to make incision of the same deade bodies for their further and better knowlage instruction in sight learnyng and experience in the sayd scyence or facultie of surgery" (Roberts and Tomlinson 1992). It was in the eighteenth century that the courts were given the power to sentence condemned prisoners to public dissection, which soon became common in Britain and most European universities (van Dijck 2005). In the United States, dissection was added to the punishment for the crimes of murder, arson, and burglary, and was sometimes designated as an alternative to gibbeting, in which the executed felon's body was caged or hung in chains and left to rot (Sappol 2002). The stigma of being sentenced to public dissection was compared to having one's body drawn and quartered, exposed, or denied burial (Carlino 1999). Denial of burial was both a disgrace and a posthumous punishment of a criminal's soul, which would not rest with the remains ungathered (Sawday 1995). Even if the mutilated remains were consigned to the cemetery after dissection, the damage had been done. The body was no longer intact, putting the afterlife of the deceased in jeopardy. On the other hand, the dissection of the body of the condemned in the service of medical science could be seen as expiation for his or her sins (Carlino 1999), and criminals who paid their dues to society were believed to avoid eternal damnation.

All the same, it was a terrifying thought to those who faced it, and a celebratory event for those who watched it. The posthumous punishment of public dissection was a show of power by the authorities, but carrying it out was sometimes — like a public execution — a rowdy and unstructured event, more akin to a lynching. Dr. A.B. Crosby of Haverhill, New Hampshire, left an account of the second half of a capital sentence being carried out on an African American man who was hanged at the turn of the nineteenth century:

> All the neighboring physicians were invited to be present and were requested to bring any dissecting instrument they might deem of use. Tradition says that one brought a hand-saw, another an axe, still another a butcher's cleaver and a fourth came armed with a large carving-knife and fork ... the cuticle of this unfortunate Ethiope was subsequently tanned and cut up into small pieces, as souvenirs ... [Washington 2006].

The regulation of dealing with the body following legal execution had the two-fold purpose of preserving the memory of the person and preventing dissection from becoming an infamous practice in the eyes of the public (Carlino 1999). More often than not, discipline was absent and neither goal was achieved.

Countless subjects of the anatomists remain anonymous, from the identities of the few dozen criminals dissected in Rome in the sixteenth century (Carlino 1999) to the name of the first American colonist to be publicly dissected, a man put to death for rape in Boston in 1734. Even though their surnames are sometimes lost to history, the fates of plenty of doubly unfortunate criminals have been recorded. In England, a murderer identified only as "Mr. Greenfield" was hanged on the infamous scaffold at Tyburn in 1689 and then pulled from his lavish coffin by chirurgeons who carried his corpse to their hall for dissection (Sawday 1995). Two criminals put to death at Newgate in 1635 were better known by their nicknames: "Canbury Bess" (Elizabeth Evans) was dissected at Surgeon's Hall and "Counterey Tom" (Thomas Shearwood) was gibbeted. After his body decayed, his skeleton was taken to Surgeon's Hall to join hers (Sawday 1995). Both Tom and Bess were notorious thieves and murderers, but often a woman was sentenced to dissection for a smaller offense than her male counterpart, because scarcer female bodies were an attraction for a mostly male audience (van Dijck 2005).

A sensational execution and dissection played out in Europe during World War I. Margaret Gertruda Zelle is better known by her stage name as an erotic dancer, Mata Hari. She found fame in Paris boasting royal

1. Anatomists as Procurers of Cadavers

Dutch and Javanese parentage, when in fact she was German. Her rivals included Isadora Duncan and her lovers were heads of European governments. But when the French, who had convinced her to spy for their country, found out that she had accepted money from a German officer, they tried her as a double agent. Accusing her of thereby causing the deaths of 50,000 soldiers, a jury sentenced her to execution by a firing squad of twelve men. She was forty-one when the sentence was carried out on October 17, 1917. Rumors flew: that her executioners wore blindfolds while she did without, that she blew them (or her lawyer) a kiss, and that she flung open her coat to reveal her nude body just before the fatal shots. Eyewitness accounts of the predawn event report that she did decline a blindfold and was dressed in a kimono, coat, hat, and gloves. Her fall to the ground was undramatic and her death was ensured with a final bullet to the temple. None of her influential former lovers came to her defense at her trial, nor did any of them — or members of her family — claim her remains or offer to pay for her burial. The body of the famous spy, which had performed so provocatively on stage, was consigned to the dissecting table at one of Paris's municipal hospitals. After she was anatomized, Mata Hari's head was embalmed and kept at the city's anatomy museum, but was later found to have disappeared.

The infamy of a criminal was as much of a draw to the general public as the occasional examination and dissection of a female body. In 1831, two men had been hanged after confessing to a murder. They had killed for the purpose of supplying the anatomists with a body, and as a punishment they were themselves dissected — an event which caused a minor riot. The public — some credentialed, some curious, and some drunk — lined up at the door to pay an entrance fee for admission to witness the dismantling of Thomas Williams (a.k.a. John Head) and John Bishop by the conservator of the Hunterian Museum, William Clift. The onlookers helped themselves to locks of hair as souvenirs and were so noisy that police had to shut down the exhibition due to complaints. After a second dissection was performed on the body of John Bishop by surgeon Richard Partridge at King's College, Cambridge, the remains were exhibited to huge crowds next to the anatomical theater. Bishop's dead body was afterward reduced to a skeleton by the medical students of the school (Wise 2004), eager to practice their techniques on any available cadaver. Clift had also anatomized the assassin of British Prime Minister Spencer Perceval, whose 1812 hanging was cheered by the crowd. Like his execution, the notorious John Bellingham's dissection was jammed with spectators. Clift opened each cavity of the body and recorded the findings, sending the stomach and left testicle to the museum. Again because cadavers were scarce, the anatomist presented the dissected body as a gift to a pupil at nearby St. Bartholomew's Hospital for further examination and anatomization (MacDonald 2005). When members of the eighteenth- and nineteenth-century American public were unable to attend public anatomy demonstrations, their curiosity could be appeased to some extent with newspaper accounts and broadsheets about the dissections of executed offenders (Sappol 2002).

Public fascination had, of course, begun hundreds of years earlier in Europe. After the fifteenth century, increased attendance at public dissections had driven anatomists to seek out the bodies of executed criminals in addition to the unclaimed dead to maintain an adequate supply of subjects. To better accommodate the audience, anatomy theaters had been erected, which — in a sort of vicious circle — often led to an increase in death row convictions (van Dijck 2005). The coarsest of criminals were consigned to the gallows, often with the additional punishment of public dissection, so this use of their bodies was generally considered appropriate and unobjectionable. Coincidentally, hanging was the preferred method of execution because it left the body with the fewest visible marks and disfigurements (van Dijck 2005, Carlino 1999). The end result of this symbiotic relationship between the condemned and the dissectors was that the public began to see both barber-surgeons and physicians as extensions of the executioner (Nunn 2005). But, like the administration of the punishment, the consignment of the bodies was most often by official decree.

In *Death, Dissection and the Destitute*, Ruth Richardson (1987) explains that the popular hostility toward dissection and the reason it was applied to the most heinous of crimes stemmed from its violation of the integrity and identity of body. In a religious sense, dissection mutilated the corpse, thereby interrupting the repose of the soul: a body that was not intact, it was believed, would not be resurrected and would have no life after death. Even though religious anatomists justified dissection as showing the hand of God in the design of the human body, it had long been associated with atheism and this couldn't be easily reconciled. On a more intellectual level, dissection causes conflict between constructs of the corpse as sacred, scientific, or saleable. And there were practical concerns. Laymen wondered whether the scraps of dissected bodies were properly buried or just eaten by beasts, as depicted in the print that they had seen reproduced, "The Rewards of Cruelty" by Hogarth. They worried about the indignities of the corpse's transport and about indecencies upon the dead bodies of women. And as punishments were carried out and the association of dissection with horrible criminals was reinforced, prejudice against dissection was perpetuated.

Allowing the public to witness the dismantling of the body amplified the horror of being dissected. As a deterrent, the coupled punishment of execution and public dissection determinedly stood for decades. After David Mylles was hanged for incest with his sister in 1703, a public dissection of his body was held in Edinburgh. In New York City, the first public anatomy in the U.S. was performed by doctors John Bard and Peter Middleton on Hermanus Carroll, who was executed in 1740. And after Thomas Grundy was hanged in Derbyshire, England, on March 29, 1788, for murdering his brother, his body was publicly dissected *in the presence of a great number of spectators.* Judges relished imposing this additional punishment and hoped it would reduce future crime. When Lord Justice Clerk pronounced sentence of death on Alexander Gillam on November 14, 1810, he ordered him hung in chains after the execution. At the same time, he expressed regret that there was no school of medicine nearby to perform a dissection, since he wanted Gillam to serve as an example. Location was less of an issue in western Scotland, where the bodies of at least twenty-three of the thirty-eight murderers hanged between 1752 and 1832 were dissected in Glasgow. And in London, the condemned were publicly dissected at Surgeon's Hall in the Old Bailey, which was conveniently adjacent to Newgate prison.

In the U.S., legislation of anatomical dissection varied by state. Virginia in 1788, for instance, refused to allow the dissection of executed criminals, but four years earlier, Massachusetts had permitted dissection not only of the bodies of criminals and the unclaimed, but the victors and victims of duels. In 1789, New York legislature passed the first law in the U.S. to sanction lawful dissection in an attempt to curb bodysnatching: An Act to Prevent the Odious Practice of Digging Up and Removing for the Purpose of Dissection Dead Bodies Buried in Cemeteries or Burial Places (Sappol 2002). By the end of the American Civil War, only Massachusetts and New York had enacted anatomy laws allowing dissection of criminals and unclaimed bodies, but the U.S. Congress later allowed judges the discretion to sentence executed criminals to dissection. By 1913, thirty-nine states had medical schools and all but five had anatomy laws. The thirty-nine states designated the use of the unclaimed dead, which were defined as bodies which were not assumed by friends or family and would require burial at public expense. Exempt were those who had requested burial, travelers who were passing through the state, and veterans. Of the states with medical schools to receive the bodies, half specified a waiting period of between ten and ninety days before allowing dissection (Shultz 1992).

In England in 1740, the surgical component of the Guild of Barber-Surgeons moved its operations from Barber's Hall to the Royal College. Shortly after their organization was professionalized, more bodies were consigned to them. In 1752, the first Anatomy Act—"An Act for better preventing the horrid Crime of Murder"—was passed by British Parliament, allowing judges the latitude to sentence the worst criminals to public dissection rather than gibbeting. Gibbeting, or hanging in chains, was intended to deny the executed felon a grave, and that further punishment was similarly extended to the dissected criminal. Disallowing the natural decay of the remains, dissection assaulted both body and soul. So to be sentenced to be hanged and publicly dissected was a mark of infamy and a fate worse than death. Carrying out the full sentence of dissection rendered the possibility of revival absolutely impossible, since this was sometimes known to happen. As examples, an Oxford woman named Anne Greene was convicted of infanticide and hanged in 1650, but regained her senses on the dissecting table of Dr. William Petty; she recovered and successfully petitioned for a pardon. Ninety years later, a seventeen-year-old thief named William Duell was hanged and allowed to swing on the gallows for half an hour, but groaned and sat up when the barber-surgeons applied the knife to his chest, after which he was banished to a penal colony instead. Dissection also sometimes revealed the "collateral damage" caused by the execution of women: when the body of Genevieve Supplice was publicly dissected by French anatomist Dr. Jean Riolan in the seventeenth century, it was found that her execution for robbery had also killed her unborn child of five months.

In the sixteenth century, the barber-surgeons in both Edinburgh and London had been allotted small numbers of bodies of executed felons by law, but almost always had to assert their granted rights by force (Sawday 1995). Similarly, after the enactment of the first Anatomy Act two hundred years later, there were often struggles — and even riots — over the bodies at the gallows. This was the case even when the beadle was present to claim bodies for the barber-surgeons. He was countered by the hangman, who had claims to the corpse's clothing, but often also trafficked in its flesh. And he was opposed by the family of the hanged criminal, who had the support of the public. Because of a riot at Tyburn, the sheriff began to take possession of the bodies of the hanged criminals and hand them over to their families unless the sentence explicitly included dissection. But he, too, could be bribed and the body confiscated by a representative of the College of Surgeons. To further complicate matters, a condemned criminal not already under sentence of dissection may have received money from an anatomist in exchange for the rights to his or her body after death. Fighting over the corpse did not necessarily end when the authority took it away in a coach: the driver was sometimes attacked and beaten so the body could be regained.

Once the corpse was in a sanctioned anatomist's custody, its confiscation was punishable by transportation for seven years. In addition to being protected by the law, the surgeons benefited from an enhanced reputation as *agents* of the law in at least one sense: by carrying out legal sentence, their status rose. They were no longer considered mere butchers, but their public esteem remained far beneath that of physicians. The surgeons still suffered from association with bodysnatchers and their task was still associated with punishment. In addition, their own motives were impugned. Not only was the association between medical men and hangmen found to be degrading, surgeons' care of their patients was questioned because of their eagerness at the gallows. They and the families of the dead were at odds because corpses were both the most valuable to anatomists and the most acutely grieved just after death. When a grave appeared to be disturbed, the home and offices of the anatomists were ransacked in an often fruitful search for the remains. Bereaved families were known to revenge the dissection of their loved ones by killing the anatomists or torching their houses.

Typical of the public anatomies of the late eighteenth and early nineteenth century, the dissections below follow well-attended executions for particularly heinous crimes. These men, many of them multiple murderers, showed no remorse for their crimes and professed to have no fear of their fate, despite the moral consequences. Their hangings were witnessed — demanded — by unsympathetic crowds. Where their victims were hidden under the bed or buried under the barn floor, their own remains were handled methodically. Their bodies were opened, examined, and experimented upon. Care was taken in order that the skulls could be assessed by phrenologists and cast to make death masks. Their bones were picked clean so that the skeletons could be harvested for the medical museum. Their skin was sent to the tannery so that books could be bound with it, shoes could be soled, and souvenirs could be distributed. The recipients of these gruesome relics were convinced that these criminals had received their just desserts: the man who killed to supply the anatomists was himself dissected, the man who split open a woman's face was opened to everyone's view on the dissecting table, and the man who cut down a family was deservedly butchered. In many cases, these hanged men, who were posthumously punished by the additional sentence of public dissection, are survived by their skeletons as well as their shared infamy.

One of the most infamous men to be publicly dissected was Sweeney Todd (1748–1802). The villainous character (and some suggest he was a creature of fiction) ran a barbershop on Fleet Street near St. Dunston's Church in London. He had learned his trade as an apprentice during a five-year stint at Newgate Prison. He became an itinerant barber upon his release at the age of nineteen, and carried out his first murder on a customer at Hyde Park Corner. When he opened his shop in London in 1785, he devised a trap door beneath the barber chair so that with the touch of a lever, he could tip his patrons into the basement. If the fall did not break the victim's neck, Todd would dispatch them with a razor to the throat. Disposing of their remains in the church crypt, Todd became the subject of speculation, but was not investigated by police.

Sometime around 1790, Todd gained the collusion of his lover Mrs. Margery (or Sarah) Lovett, a widow and local baker in Bell Yard. An underground passage between the two establishments allowed the flesh of the victims to be transferred to Mrs. Lovett's shop for inclusion in the meat pies for which she was known. The butchering of the bodies was carried out by Todd after he stripped the valuables from the body and removed the deceased's clothing. Working quickly to avoid the problems associated with rigor mortis, the barber would cut the limbs off at the joints. The skin would be removed and discarded, since it would have been detectable in the pies. Then, by the flickering light of his oil lamps and candles, Todd would disembowel his victims. He would strip all of the flesh from the bones and grind up the vital organs to yield even more meat for the pies. He boxed the fresh meat for delivery to his partner in crime. The bones were casually scattered amid the unburied remains in the catacombs, where they were virtually indistinguishable from the bodies of persons who had died more natural deaths. But by 1800, the stench from the crypt at St. Dunston's drew investigation by the church beadle and the police chief. The remains of a supposed 160 victims were discovered, bloody footprints led to the bakery, and both Todd and Lovett were arrested. Mrs. Lovett made a full confession, then took poison and died.

Todd was tried for the murder of a single man, seaman Richard Thornhill, which his defense tried to pin on Mrs. Lovett. Dr. Sylvester Steers was called upon to identify Thornhill's remains, in what is said to be the first use of forensic evidence in court:

> Mr. Thornhill met with a very unusual and painful accident.... The external condyle or projection on the outer end of the thighbone, which makes part of the knee joint, was broken off, and there was a diagonal fracture about three inches higher upon the bone. I had the sole care of the case, and although a cure was effected, it was not without considerable distortion of the bone. From my frequent examination I was perfectly well acquainted with the case, and I can swear that the bone in the hands of the jury was the one so broken to which I attended [Gribben n.d.].

The jury deliberated for a mere five minutes before sentencing Todd to the gallows. On January 25, 1802, Sweeney Todd was hanged from the gallows of Newgate Prison, where he had been incarcerated as an adolescent. After the execution, Todd's body was dissected as part of his punishment.

Sweeney Todd's story first appeared in a mid-nineteenth century penny dreadful and has since been told in films, on the stage, and in song. Its veracity has been challenged by scholars, who find no record of his trial in December 1801 or his execution in January 1802. Nevertheless, the dubious facts of Todd's demise are as follows. The judge placed a black cloth on top of his white wig to pronounce sentence. Asked if he had any words, Todd shouted, "I am not guilty!" The judge then sentenced him to be taken to the place of execution and hanged by the neck until dead, adding, "May Heaven have mercy upon you. You cannot expect that society can do otherwise than put out of life someone who, like yourself, has been a terror and a scourge" (Gribben n.d.). Todd was hanged in the prison yard at Newgate before a crowd of thousands, some of whom reported that he "died hard." Afterward, his body was released to barber-surgeons, who dissected it, a fate many found fitting. Whether or not the story of Sweeney Todd is truth or merely legend, it demonstrates the pattern established by the first Anatomy Act, under which executed felons gave up not only their lives but their bodies to the State.

In the year 1832, British parliament passed the Second Anatomy Act. Among many administrative clauses was a momentous change in the law. The Act abolished the use of dissection as a punishment for murder. Instead it compelled the release to anatomists of unclaimed bodies from workhouses, hospitals, charitable institutions, prisons, and places of public charge. It contained no guidelines governing the retention of skeletons and specimens removed from the anatomized bodies. With the passage of this Second Anatomy Act, the government replaced the bodies of criminals in the anatomy theater with the bodies of the poor. Those unfortunate enough to die in the poorhouse and — because claiming a body meant taking responsibility for the funeral expenses — those who could not afford to bury their loved ones were the victims of discrimination. The Act punished the impoverished, and the poor were understandably outraged. They feared that the members of their class would be butchered, that cholera victims would receive minimal care, and that the second Act — like the first — was being used retributively.

One of the first examples that the Second Anatomy Act was being applied punitively occurred in December 1832. Mary Ann "Polly" Chapman — a known prostitute — drowned herself in the London Dock, distraught that she couldn't pay her rent. She had been destitute, so her body was given over to London Hospital for dissection. But because the authorities wanted to make an example of her, they denied the request of her fellow prostitutes to claim and bury her body. Although this Second Anatomy Act ensured a legal supply of bodies, the procurement of the dead by the anatomists was still fraught with mistakes and misconceptions. Members of the lower class did whatever they could to avoid entering the workhouse, aware of their likely fate if they died. But at the same time, the Act did not anticipate that anyone would *voluntarily* donate his or her body for dissection, so one of the first opportunities to encourage this selfless act was squandered. When Peter Baume delivered the bodies of his sister Charlotte and her baby to the anatomy school at London University — as she had requested before their deaths in December 1832 — he was promptly arrested on suspicion of murder, and only later cleared without apology.

The application of the Second Anatomy Act also lacked in other ways. For one thing, hospital schools of anatomy had an advantage because they received bodies from their own morgues. Members of the medical profession were eager to gain respect by severing their relationship with the hangman, yet maintained their ties with the so-called "resurrectionists." Bodysnatching alone had produced only a slightly smaller number of subjects than the five hundred per year that were delivered for dissection in the London area in the first decade after the passage of the Anatomy Act. The transfer of bodies was still done covertly and the details were kept from general public knowledge. Tuition fees were not adjusted downward to take into consideration the legal supply of subjects for anatomy classes. Bodies were wrongfully dissected. And corruption still flourished, with gravediggers accepting both payment from the family for burying the coffin and another sum to deliver the intended contents to the anatomy laboratory.

Bodysnatching had begun in Britain in the seventeenth century to fill the demand for bodies to dissect that was not met by the gallows or the poorhouse. Teachers of anatomy had pressed anatomical models into service, and had learned how best to preserve specimens for reuse, but

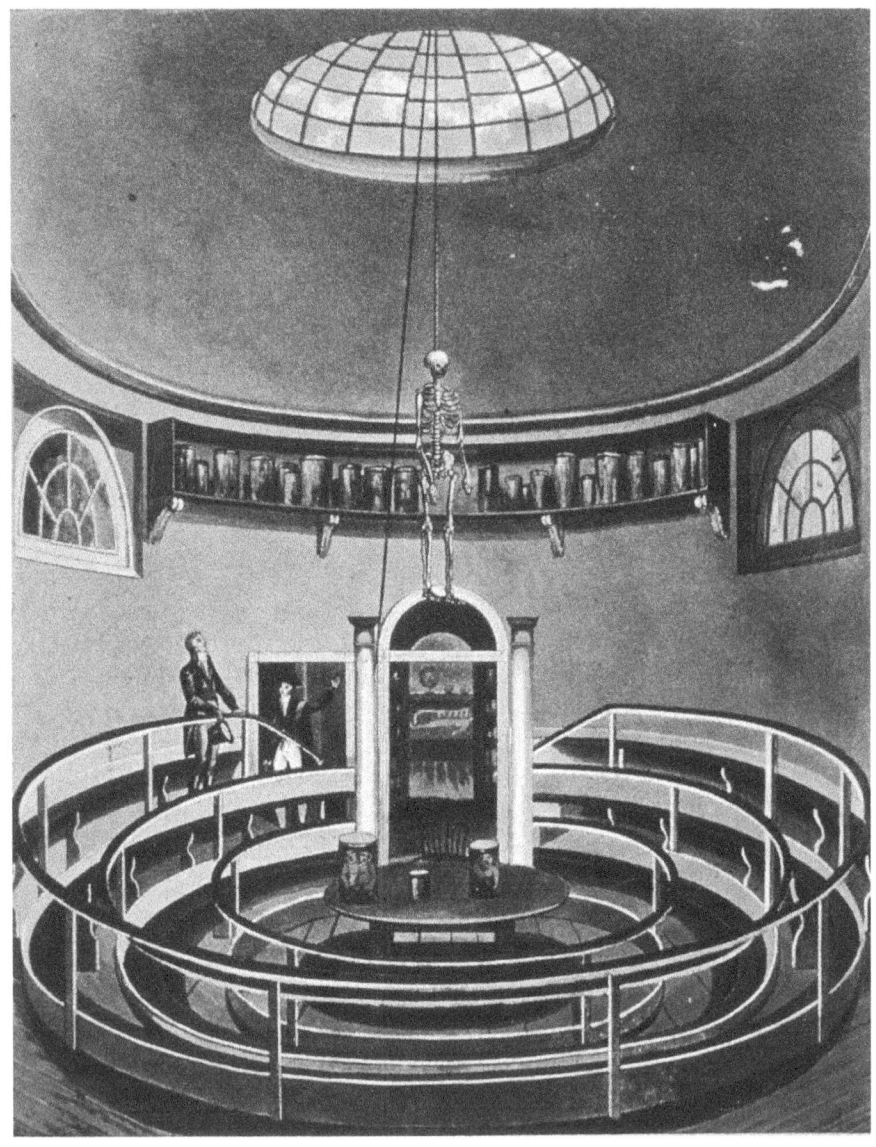

This 1815 print shows an anatomical theater in London with windows and a skylight to provide natural light. A skeleton is suspended in the center and wet specimens line a shelf. Like the two visitors to the empty theater, observers of a dissection would have stood at the railings (*courtesy National Library of Medicine*).

1. Anatomists as Procurers of Cadavers

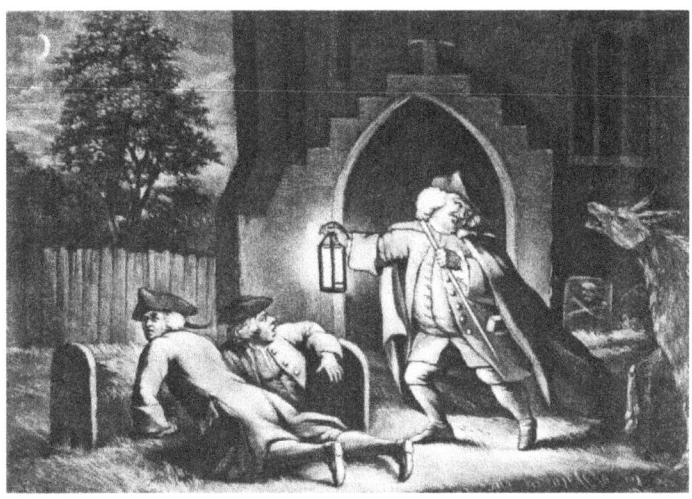

In this 1771 mezzotint, bodysnatchers have been startled by an ass as they work under cover of darkness in St. Paul's churchyard to disinter a recently buried body for the purpose of supplying it to an anatomist for dissection (*Wellcome Images*).

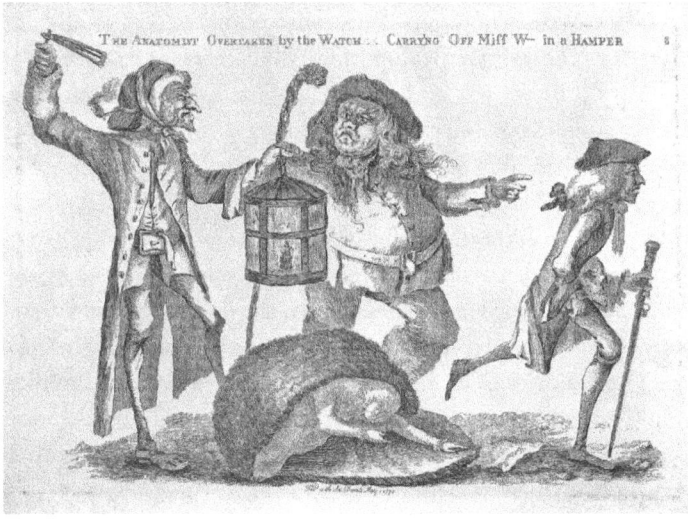

A 1773 etching caricatures anatomist William Hunter, who runs away from the scene as a resurrectionist is caught transporting a fresh corpse from the cemetery in a hamper by a nightwatchman. Bodies were sold for dissection based on their length (*Wellcome Images*).

found that there was no substitute for a fresh cadaver. Anatomists, desperate for bodies on which to train their students, robbed the graveyards of their recent dead, or compelled their students to do so. Some professors would even accept bodies from their students in lieu of tuition. The scarcity of bodies drove students to the cities of London and Paris to study anatomy, and kept this illicit trade alive in the United Kingdom until the 1850s and in the United States until 1930—only waning as embalming gained popularity and dissecting didn't require such immediacy. Early on, anatomists had delegated the gruesome and illegal task of procuring buried bodies to middlemen. Resurrectionists would do the dirty work of exhuming fresh bodies from their graves to sell to the anatomists. The corpse was often disrobed and the clothes left behind, because stealing the grave goods was the felony—except in Scotland, where bodysnatchers were charged with "violating the sepulchres of the dead."

Bodysnatchers worked in pairs or gangs and quickly learned how to exhume bodies most efficiently—by digging up only half the grave, snapping the coffin lid in half, and hauling out the corpse by means of a rope tied under the shoulders. But resurrectionists William Burke (discussed below) and his partner in crime William Hare discovered that it was less work if burial was eliminated altogether. When a lodger in their boarding house died owing them money, they sold his body for dissection to settle the debt. This led Burke and Hare to carry out more than a dozen murders for the prices they could obtain for such fresh subjects. Careful not to mutilate the bodies in the process, the killings were done by smothering, and the newly coined word "burking" entered the language to describe their method. Similarly, the eponyms "Burkimania" or "Burkiphobia" were used to describe the fear of being murdered for dissection. The majority of bodies that were snatched belonged to the poor, who could not afford to post guards or install contraptions like mortsafes to protect graves. Consequently, the lower classes soon realized that their bodies were worth more dead than alive. Prostitutes, vagrants, and the occasional bodysnatcher took advantage of this by pre-selling the rights to their own bodies after death.

The numbers are staggering. In early nineteenth-century London, when the whole city was invited to attend dissections, a total of ten bodysnatchers were regularly employed, and yet they could not sufficiently supply the medical school in the city's West End, which closed along with schools in Sheffield, Bristol, Liverpool, and Manchester due to a lack of cadavers (Lassek 1958). At the same time, the schools in England and Scotland were importing thousands of bodies from Dublin, where resurrectionists were pulling corpses by the hundreds from a single potter's field called Bully's Acre (Lassek 1958). Similarly in the American states, Case Western Reserve University was importing bodies — most of them African American — from Virginia, Tennessee, Georgia, Alabama, Kentucky, Arkansas, and North and South Carolina. African Americans saw dissection as an extension of slavery, representing white control over their bodies that kept them from being free, in death as in life. Even when the bodysnatcher was black, as in the case of a man commissioned by Jefferson Medical College in Philadelphia to deliver bodies from the local African American cemetery, they lay the blame squarely at the feet of white physicians (Washington 2006).

African American oral tradition holds that the bodies of their dead have been stolen by "night doctors" under the cover of darkness for medical dissection or use in laboratories, and this is not far from the truth. Their bodies have been disproportionately used to teach anatomy in schools to the north and to the south. The Medical College of Georgia obtained subjects that had been stolen from Cedar Grove Cemetery, the African American burial ground established after the Civil War. Both New York University and Columbia University procured most of the cadavers they needed for their classes from the Negro Burying Ground. Before emancipation, slave-owners who sent sick slaves to the hospital promised their bodies to the institution in exchange for caring for them. After slavery was abolished, hospitals expected blacks who had been treated in the charity wards to submit to autopsy and dissection after their deaths (Washington 2006). As a symbol of the domination of African Americans in the U.S., and more widely as half of a punishment reserved for the most notorious criminals, dissection was looked upon as shameful and disgusting. Those whose illegal activities helped propel it were equally abhorrent.

Bodysnatchers had no respect for the sanctity of the graves they disturbed, nor apparently for each other. One named Ben Crouch repeatedly embezzled money from the treasury of his own gang, using his prowess as a former prizefighter to squelch any objection. They guarded their methods from newcomers attempting to break into the profession, as described in the nineteenth-century biography of English anatomist Sir Astley Cooper:

> Another motive for their strict secresy as to their method of working, was, that their band, which consisted of considerably fewer persons than was generally supposed, might not be disturbed by the intrusive entry of fresh men, who, in the hope of obtaining their share of the great profit derived from such occupation, were not unfrequently attempting to invade what the Resurrectionists almost thought to be their exclusive right of trade. As, on the one hand, it was the object of the party seeking admission into this business, to discover the peculiar method by which the initiated accomplished their objects, so rapidly, and, in proportion with diminished risk; so, on the other hand, it was the object of the monopolizers, by throwing a mystery around their mode of working, to prevent this discovery taking place; and further to secure themselves against such an event they would endeavour to set the new comers on a wrong scent, and so lead to their detection [Cooper 1843].

The bodysnatchers did form gangs, although a few among them took leadership roles.

William Cunningham (1807–1871) is perhaps the most famous American bodysnatcher, and was reviled during his lifetime. His contemporaries called him "Old Man Dead" or "The Ghoul," but he was better known as "Old Cunny" because of his name and his cunning escapades. These were carried out at night, between the years of 1855 and 1871. During the day, the strong and hard-drinking Irishman worked as a drayman transporting legitimate goods. But his horse and wagon served another purpose as he spent his nights procuring "anatomical material" for the professors of the medical colleges of Cincinnati, Ohio. One of Old Cunny's clients described his transport method:

> Usually he took the body to town in a buggy sitting in the seat beside him. The corpse was dressed up in an old coat, vest and hat. He would hold the reins in his right hand while he would steady the corpse with his left arm around the waist of his silent companion. Whenever people passed and the corpse would gravitate forward and

downward Cunny would slap his inoffensive partner in the face and say to him, "Sit up! This is the last time I am going to take you home when you get drunk. The idea of a man with a family disgracing himself in this way!" [Edwards 1955].

Cunningham was held in high regard by the medical men who depended on his black market services, but was viewed with suspicion by the other members of the community.

In one well-remembered incident, Cunny and two hired helpers stopped at a Carthage saloon in the hour before midnight. They then proceeded to the cemetery in the rear of the City Infirmary. Uncertain of their intentions, the rest of the establishment's patrons formed a posse and followed them. When the posse reached the cemetery, they found Cunny and his confederates raising two subjects from their graves, so they surrounded the bodysnatchers and began firing indiscriminately. The hired hands fled into the woods, but Cunny stood his ground until a rifle pointed directly at him misfired. He was begging for his life when they took him into custody and forced him to drive his wagon back to Carthage, but by the time they had returned to the village he had persuaded his captors to stop again at the saloon. After he plied them with several rounds of drinks, they allowed him to return to Cincinnati with his empty wagon. But instead of going home, he circled back to the cemetery where his dutiful helpers awaited him with the two bodies already sacked up for transport.

On another occasion, Cunny and two helpers were caught with two bodies they had just disinterred from a cemetery near Hartley, Ohio. The men were arrested and taken to the police station, and the bodies were delivered to a nearby funeral home for identification. After a night in jail, the bodysnatchers were released on bail. That afternoon, two men passed themselves off as officials from the coroner's office and demanded that the funeral director's assistant relinquish the bodies so that an inquest could be held. This was, of course, a ruse and the officials had neither sent for nor seen the bodies. Without them as evidence of a crime, Cunny and company could not be charged. Neither was a "rival gang" charged for stealing a cadaver Cunningham had delivered to a medical college himself. Cunny complained of the burden of having to make another midnight run to replace it, when in fact he may have stolen the body himself and sold it to a rival institution, thereby tripling his profits!

Not only did Cunningham deliver in person, he apparently offered mail order, as postal agents found out in 1870 when they opened a C.O.D. parcel he had dropped off at the U.S. express office. The box never made it to its destination — Dr. M.P. Hayden, Leavenworth, Kansas — because opening it revealed the dissection-ready body of an African American woman. Cunny took no revenge on the post office, which returned the freight to him, but he was known to have paid back some medical students for an unrecorded prank they played on him. He deliberately supplied them with a smallpox victim for their next dissection, an act of retaliation that caused a number of them to fall sick.

It can be assumed from stories in the Cincinnati newspapers of the day that William Cunningham made a good living as a bodysnatcher. One story notes that upon an arrest for public drunkenness he was found with the large sum of $70 in his pocket, and another story alludes to his purchase of a brand new $400 carriage. But the August 31, 1871, edition of the *Cincinnati Daily Gazette* reported that his career had finally come to an end. After years of escaping punishment, his age — and the law — had finally caught up to him. He was driving down the street at a great rate of speed, being chased by a crowd of men and boys shouting, "Stop him! Shoot him!" The spectacle drew the attention of two police officers, who were able to catch up with him and grab the horse's bridle when Cunny refused their orders to stop. The dray was in fact lame and the wagon had sustained an accident on the way home from his night's work. The mob had discovered, and the police confirmed, that he had the bodies of an adult man and an eleven- or twelve-year-old boy on board.

Cunningham was arrested and indicted on five counts of illegal possession of dead human bodies. He was released on $300 bail and ordered to answer to the charges at the next session of the Common Pleas Court. Although it is unknown whether he appeared, a subsequent issue of the *Cincinnati Daily Enquirer* places him as a patient in the Cincinnati Hospital, where he was suffering from the effects of rotgut whiskey, and promising to be back in business in a matter of days. But on November 2, 1871, Old Cunny died of heart trouble at the age of 64. Before his demise, however, he had sold his own body to the Medical College of Ohio. His corpse was delivered to that institution by his widow, who received an additional $5 for it (and for a time reportedly carried on his ghoulish livelihood). After Cunny's cadaver was dissected, his skeleton was harvested and placed on display in the college's museum, after which it passed into the collections of the Department of Anatomy of the College of Medicine at the University of Cincinnati.

Old Cunny's skeleton was visited at the museum by an African American man who sometimes worked for him. "To him there was nothing more in the handling of bodies than in so many bolts of cloth or sacks of grain, and no more in dissection than in the business of the butcher or the meat-vendor," reads the *New York Times* ("He stands by his trade" 1878). Charley Keaton was moved by Cunningham's example to sell his own body after death to the Medical College of Ohio, thus furthering the study of anatomy and gaining him an immediate $35. Upon his death in 1878 at the approximate age of forty, Keaton's corpse was — without the usual secrecy — taken from the wagon, carried up the stairs to the "dead-room," and unclothed. His remains had previously been prepared by his wife, who had often accompanied him on his nightly excursions, and funeralized at home by his family. His blood was drained and a preservative fluid was injected into the arteries, after which his body was added to more than a dozen others in the pickling bath. Keaton, having worked as a bodysnatcher until a few short weeks before his own death, had demonstrated his desire for his remains to be dissected in the interest of science rather than decay underground in Potter's Field. And he had expressed an interest in keeping Old Cunny company when his skeleton joined that of the infamous old man.

While the occasional resurrectionist may have pledged his remains to the anatomist, pairing medical dissection with punishment and illegal activity did voluntary body donation a disservice. Dissected felons were considered to have made a sort of reparation to fellow humans by becoming useful after death, but the cloud of dishonor hung over innocent donors who wanted the use of their bodies to benefit society. Anatomists, associated with wrangling bodies from the ground, from the gallows, and even — by prepayment — from condemned men not already under sentence of dissection, were caught in the middle. They were accused by the public of being hypocrites by not setting the example and donating their own bodies. William Hunter, for instance, insisted that his body be wrapped in lead upon his death to thwart fellow anatomists. Almost fifty years later, the example was instead set by English philosopher and social reformer Jeremy Bentham, who was dissected after death at his own request. As instructed, close friend and fellow utilitarian Dr. Southwood Smith conducted a public dissection on Bentham's body three days after death to illustrate "the Structures and Functions of the Human Frame," as it said on the printed invitations. On June 9, 1832, at his anatomy school in Southwark, London, Dr. Smith's lecture over the body "on the Usefulness of Knowledge of this kind to the Community" addressed the importance of his principles over his personal feelings: "If, by any appropriation of the dead, I can promote the happiness of the living, then it is my duty to conquer the reluctance I may feel to such a disposition of the dead, however well-founded or strong that reluctance may be."

Dissection did not preclude Bentham's funeralization or memorialization: mourning rings were distributed afterward, and an "auto-icon" was prepared from his remains to obviate the need to commission a sculpture. The skeleton was padded and dressed in his customary clothes, topped by his mummified head (later replaced with a wax portrait). This was placed in a seated position in a glass-fronted cabinet which sat in Dr. Smith's office until donated to University College London, where it still resides. Bentham's example of philanthropic body donation was followed by the Duke of Sussex, who gave orders that his corpse should be given to students for dissection the same year that Bentham was anatomized. Prominent Boston physician J.C. Warren also had his body publicly dissected before a respectful professional assembly, but such acts remained exceptional (Sappol 2002). It wasn't until after World War II — and in correspondence with increased atheism and cremation — that whole-body donation levels rose above 70 percent of all dissections.

One man who was absolutely opposed to donating his body to science was the eighteenth-century giant Charles Byrne, knowing that his dramatic height made his corpse a prize. And the one man determined to have his bones was John Hunter, an anatomist so prolific that he was a favorite client of the local bodysnatchers. With discretion, Hunter was able to obtain even the bodies of pregnant women, which he dissected to illustrate his text about the gravid uterus. With bribery, Hunter was able to secure Byrne's body in spite of the precautions the man had taken in advance of his death to avoid just such a fate. Long before having to adhere to the doctrine of obtaining informed consent, Hunter was boiling the bones of the oversize skeleton in his basement. An enthusiastic dissector, Sir Astley Cooper was also on good terms with the bodysnatchers, and was able to obtain — through them — the bodies of specific patients he wanted to examine. Cooper educated his students in the fine points of anatomy, but also demanded that they participate in the rougher art of lifting their subjects from their graves. Cooper, like his colleagues, was forced to turn to the cemeteries for material, since the need for fresh corpses to dissect far outstripped the number that were provided to them legally. He shared this insight into London's postmortem economics with a parliamentary committee, noting that cracking down on the robbing of graves only raises the price of the bodies — and informing their decision to enact the Second Anatomy Act.

There is irony in the fact that eighteenth-century Edinburgh anatomist Alexander Monro primus resorted to patronizing bodysnatchers. These reviled men, who by definition desecrated the sacred space of the cemetery and disturbed the eternal slumber of the dead, obtained by immoral means the cadavers on which to demonstrate their wondrous workings at the hand of the ingenius Creator. These bodies would have been in the early stages of decomposition, so the Monro patriarch saw fit during dissection to draw the attention of his students to the area upon which they would concentrate by adding color to the pallid corpse. Monro's youngest son, distinguished as Alexander Monro secundus, was groomed to be his successor and took his place alongside his father at the dissecting table at a young age. This immersion in the field of anatomy, especially at its center of Edinburgh during the 1800s, would have ensured the necessary training in the barter with the bodysnatchers. It had all become rather routine by the time the third-generation Monro took over the post. Alexander Monro tertius is remembered as grubby and dull, qualities that caused students to gravitate to his rival. Dr. Knox's teaching style required a greater supply of bodies, which worked indirectly to Monro's advantage. Monro gained lasting fame not for the quality of the dissections he carried on in the family name, but for the anatomization of one of Knox's notorious suppliers.

The resurrectionists collected the bodies from which the anatomists collected their specimens, in addition to instructing their students and informing their own studies. Monro primus ran out of room to store his anatomical preparations and had to lobby the university for more space, which he was soon given. John Hunter offered the vast collection he had amassed over his lifetime — thousands of specimens, some of which he had expertly prepared, and others of which he had acquired — to the British government. The Hunterian collection was finally purchased, although the catalog meticulously kept by its namesake had been destroyed in a fit of jealousy and the greater part of the original specimens — Byrne's skeleton excepted — was later destroyed in an act of war. And it was contemporary conflict, the Napoleonic wars, that prompted Astley Cooper to prepare the specimen still on display at Guy's Hospital: the famous example of an experimental ligation of the abdominal aorta. After the bodysnatchers disturbed the eternal repose of the dead, the anatomists offered them a peculiar and often nameless immortality.

Alexander Monro Primus (1697–1767) and His Legacy

The Monro dynasty held the Edinburgh anatomy chair for a total of 126 years. Patriarch Alexander Monro primus studied in Scotland, England, France, and the Netherlands before returning to Edinburgh to teach. In London he participated in a two-month course consisting of thirty-five lectures by William Cheselden (discussed below). Monro primus read, learned to prepare specimens, and dissecting plenty of human bodies — no doubt acquired by graverobbing — with several colleagues, including Scottish physicians James Douglas and William Rutty. Monro stayed in Paris for several months, attending a course in anatomy and surgery at the Hotel-Dieu and public lectures in chemistry, anatomy, and botany at the Jardin du Roi. He then rounded out his education by spending a year in the anatomical center of Leiden, during which time he met Amsterdam anatomist Frederik Ruysch and attended classes in medicine and chemistry taught by renowned Dutch physician Hermann Boerhaave. He observed the public dissections carried out in the anatom-

1. Anatomists as Procurers of Cadavers (Alexander Monro Primus)

ical theater founded in 1597 by Pieter Paaw, the first professor of anatomy at the University of Leiden.

Back in his home country, Monro primus performed public dissections of his own. He had been appointed professor of anatomy at the University of Edinburgh in 1720 on the recommendation of the Edinburgh Incorporation of Surgeons, to which he had been admitted the previous year. Like other anatomists of the time, he demonstrated on animals as stand-ins for humans. But once a year he was responsible for the public dissection of a human body, a duty that had been carried out only intermittently since its inception in 1697. The dissections were carried out in Surgeon's Hall, in which he probably housed his wet specimens until he was provided with a lecture room at the University. He complained that the room, the floor of which was below ground level, never admitted enough light and did not have sufficient room for his anatomical preparations, and he lobbied for a new anatomy theater that was built in 1725. Monro had begun a course on anatomy consisting of more than one hundred lectures that, within two decades, attracted 150 students each year.

Monro primus's lectures were lively, anecdotal, and delivered without referring to notes. He supplemented human dissection with demonstrations on wet specimens, experiments on animals, and examinations under the microscope. He endeavored to make his cadavers aesthetically pleasing by accentuating the area of focus by adding some natural color and using a flap of skin from the abdominal dissection to cover the genitals. In preparing skeletal displays, he strove for whiteness and smoothness. Monro's demonstrations were as much about natural theology as they were about anatomy, though his lecture room was not decorated with moral lessons like the Leiden theater. Nevertheless, his dissections were not merely meant to unravel the human body to teach would-be surgeons, but to show by its internal workings that the body was the ingenious creation of God. His style of teaching anatomy as part of a philosophical curriculum was typical of the so-called "Scottish method" that held sway until anatomists began to incorporate a more mechanical mindset.

Alexander Monro primus had chosen his third and youngest son, born in 1733, to follow him in his profession. He saw that the boy received a solid education, and allowed Alexander Monro secundus to take up a scalpel when he showed an inclination for anatomy at an early age. By the age of eighteen, the boy had embarked on his medical career and was assisting his father in the dissecting room. In 1753, when the size of his class exceeded the size of his lecture hall and Alexander Monro primus found himself giving two identical lectures a day, he allowed his son to take over the evening lectures. He appealed to the Edinburgh Town Council to name Alexander Monro secundus as his successor, and shortly thereafter the young man was admitted to the University faculty. He took his degree as Doctor of Medicine in 1775 and then — like his father — continued his education in London, Paris, and Leiden. But unlike his father, Alexander Monro secundus concentrated his studies abroad in Berlin. He returned to Edinburgh first to fill in for his father who had been taken ill and then, after being admitted to the Royal College of Surgeons of Edinburgh, to take over for him completely.

Alexander Monro tertius, too, studied in London and Paris (though not Leiden), then returned to Edinburgh, where he served jointly on the faculty with his father. He taught the entire course beginning in 1808, and became sole professor in 1817. But by the time he followed in the footsteps of his father and grandfather, Edinburgh University's reputation had declined and the appointment of its professors had more to do with politics than with ability. Though he had in essence inherited the anatomy chair, the third-generation Alexander Monro did not rank with the earlier Monros and added little original material to the lecture notes he inherited from them. Alexander Monro tertius was considered an uninspired, indifferent, and mediocre teacher. One of his students in 1825, Charles Darwin, disliked his lectures and dirty personal habits so much that he turned from surgery to natural history. Darwin was known to have called Monro's lectures on human anatomy as dull as he was himself. Other students transferred to competing private schools, including that established in 1826 by Robert Knox. Knox educated his students in the Parisian manner, which called for more corpses on which to demonstrate anatomy. He turned to bodysnatchers Burke and Hare to procure them, a decision that resulted in the public dissection for which Alexander Monro tertius is best known.

William Burke and his partner in crime William Hare are perhaps

1. Anatomists as Procurers of Cadavers (Alexander Monro Primus)

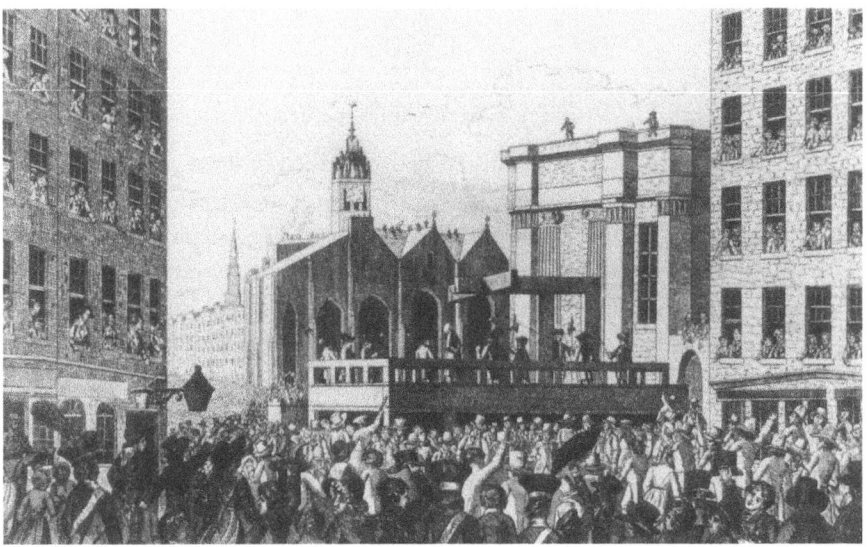

An 1829 lithograph used in a book illustration depicts the crowds present at the hanging of notorious Scottish bodysnatcher William Burke, who supplied Dr. Knox with subjects. Burke had the help of his accomplice William Hare, whose life was spared in exchange for turning Queen's evidence, but it is "burking" that has became eponymous with killing to sell the body of the victim for medical dissection. Burke's sentence fittingly included the dissection of his own body. Burke's skeleton was sent to the Royal College of Surgeons of Edinburgh, and souvenirs were crafted from his skin (*courtesy National Library of Medicine*).

history's most notorious bodysnatchers. The two met when Burke and his mistress moved into a lodging house run by Hare and his common-law wife in Edinburgh in 1827. Shortly thereafter, a fellow lodger died owing them money. To settle the debt, they decided to sell his body for dissection. After making inquiries, they offered the corpse to Dr. Robert Knox and received £7 for it with "no questions asked" regarding its freshness. This transaction convinced them that producing corpses would be easier and more lucrative than stealing them from their graves. Over the ensuing months, they killed several people, including another tenant, two old women, two prostitutes, a beggar woman, and a deaf boy. Due to the method they used, so as not to mutilate their victims, "burking" entered the language as a synonym for smothering. In addition, the following rhyme became part of the repertoire of Scottish schoolchildren:

> Up the close and doon the stair,
> "But an' ben wi" Burke an' Hare,
> Burke's the butcher, Hare's the thief,
> Knox the man that buys the beef.

Burke and Hare are believed to have killed at least sixteen people over an eighteen-month period, taking greater and greater risks — like murdering a popular street entertainer named "Daft Jamie," who was recognized on the dissecting table because of his deformed foot. But the befriending of a Mrs. Docherty in a local shop led to their undoing. Luring her back to their lodging house, they smothered her and deposited her body under a bed. Fellow lodgers became suspicious and, despite bribes to keep quiet, reported their concerns to police. Bruke and Hare were arrested and the body of Mrs. Docherty was found in Dr. Knox's classroom. Their complicit wives were also arrested, but were not prosecuted and fled the country for fear of being lynched. Despite a public uproar, no charges were brought against Dr. Knox, but his career suffered greatly.

Burke and Hare were put on trial, but with scant evidence against them. Hare was offered immunity from prosecution for his testimony and was released, with little known for sure about the rest of his life. Burke, on the other hand, was convicted by the court. The handbill describing his sentencing and execution reads, "Burke's body is to be dissected, and his Skeleton to be preserved, in order that posterity may keep in remembrance his atrocious crimes." He readily admitted to his crimes during his weeks of incarceration and prayed with a number of spiritual advisors. Anxious about his fate, though remaining calm, he was quoted by the newspapers as saying, "Oh that the hour has come which is to separate me from this world." He thanked everyone for their consolation and kindness, except for the executioner, to whom he remarked, "I am not just ready for you yet." The day before the execution, workmen assembled the gibbet at the Lawnmarket in Edinburgh and erected a barrier to hold back the crowd, which had already begun to gather even in the pouring rain — and later let out three cheers when the job was completed. Burke, pale and dressed in black, arrived at the gallows on the morning of January 28, 1829. The crowd of at least 20,000, some of whom had paid for views from the windows of local establishments, erupted in a shout. The noise subsided as final prayers were offered for the prisoner, then resumed with cheers, groans, and hisses. As the executioner positioned the rope, drew the cloth over his face, and placed the signal in the prisoner's hand, the crowd cried, "Burke him. Do the same for Hare." Burke uttered a prayer, signaled, and the drop fell. The lively crowd cheered again at every convulsive movement, but his agony did not last long and his body was cut down within the hour. A final cry erupted before the crowd dispersed.

Upon the earlier recommendation of the judge, Burke's body was destined for dissection — although researcher Ruth Richardson has found that Burke had no fear of this fate. Fittingly, Burke's remains were conveyed overnight to the classroom of Dr. Alexander Monro tertius, Dr. Knox's rival at the Edinburgh Medical College, who lectured upon the brain to his students the following day. Dipping his quill pen into Burke's blood, Monro wrote, "This is written with the blood of Wm Burke, who was hanged at Edinburgh. This blood was taken from his head." A crowd said to number 2,000 assembled at the door, demanding entrance and rioting against the police. After Monro's lecture was concluded, they were allowed to enter and file past Burke's corpse. The next day, an even larger crowd appeared at the college gates, so the doors to the hall were thrown open to the public and the newspaper described the sight:

> The corpse was stretched on the dissecting table in a state of nudity, and although the skull had been taken off on the previous day, to allow the lecturer to expose the brain, the eyes were more than half open, quite bright, and the features were so little distorted, that they were instantly recognised by numbers to whom he had been previously unknown by name.... The corpse lay exposed for seven hours and a half and it is utterly impossible to say at what period the pressure was most severe. The progress of this "stream of people" was slow but constant, and yesterday the body was seen by upwards of 24,000 individuals.

Burke's skeleton was retained and is still on display in the Anatomy Museum at Edinburgh University. His death mask and a wallet stamped with the words "Burke's Skin Pocket Book" are preserved in the Surgeon's Hall Museum of the Royal College of Surgeons in Edinburgh. A small gold-embossed business card case made from the skin of his left hand is exhibited in Edinburgh's Police Museum and a small piece of his skin can be seen in the Smith Art Gallery and Museum in Stirling. Other items crafted from Burke's skin are believed to be in private collections.

William Burke was not the only notorious criminal to be dissected by the third Alexander Monro. John Howison became known as the "Cramond Murderer" after he was accused of a particularly gruesome murder in which an elderly woman's face had been split open with a spade in her own home. He was arrested the day after the murder, although he resisted arrest by police and claimed innocence by virtue of the fact that no one had witnessed the crime. Howison was brought to trial by the end of the month and a verdict of guilty of murder was unanimously rendered in a matter of days. His sentence — to be hanged and dissected — was the last of its kind in the U.K. before the implementation of the Anatomy Act of 1832. Accordingly, he was executed in Edinburgh on Saturday, January 21, 1832, then taken from the gallows and given over to Dr. Munro of Edinburgh University to be anatomized. A broadside about his execution describes the scene.

> He appeared on the scaffold shortly after eight, where he remained but for a short time, and while a most devout prayer was offered for him to the Throne of Grace for mercy. All things being prepared, he mounted the fatal drop; and, after a few minutes, he reluctantly dropped the signal, and was instantly launched into eternity. He was about 44 years of age, of very loathsome and uncouth appearance. After hanging the usual time, the body was cut down, and sent to the College for dissection.

Howison's skeleton was preserved and now shares a display case with that of notorious body-snatcher William Burke in Edinburgh University's Anatomy Museum. Alexander Monro retired in 1846 and died in 1859, ending the Monro dynasty with historical notoriety rather than high regard by his students and peers.

John Hunter (1728–1793) and His Brother

Anatomist John Hunter professed to have dissected thousands of human bodies during his career. Known for his dexterity, he had learned

1. Anatomists as Procurers of Cadavers (John Hunter)

to handle knives and saws with precision while working in his brother-in-law's timber yard. He left Scotland for the first time in 1748 and performed his first dissection under his brother William's watchful eye in London. William's newly-established anatomy school — the first of its kind in Great Britain — was due to begin the Fall term in two weeks. William, ten years John's senior, had studied under Alexander Munro primus at Edinburgh University and found the anatomy demonstrations wanting: "There I learned a good deal by my ears; but almost nothing by my eyes; and therefore, hardly anything to the purpose. The defect was, that the professor was obliged to demonstrate all the parts of the body, except the bones, nerves, and vessels, upon one dead body" (Moore 2005). A mere two corpses were used during a series of thirty-nine lectures he attended in London. Having witnessed the more plentiful use of bodies for dissection in Paris and Leiden, Hunter was determined that his school would fill the void for London's would-be anatomists.

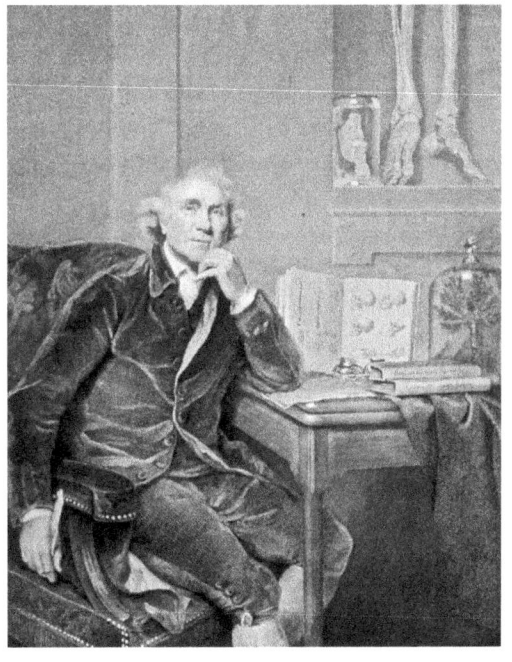

This 18th century portrait by Sir Joshua Reynolds depicts Scottish anatomist John Hunter seated and surrounded by textbooks and specimens, including the skeleton of the Irish giant Charles Byrne, which Hunter obtained illicitly and against Byrne's wishes (*courtesy National Library of Medicine*).

William rented an apartment in Covent Garden to house a lecture theater and dissecting room and advertised this new opportunity to learn the art of dissection in the Parisian manner, in which each pupil dissected a cadaver of his own. The courses William offered included seventy lessons over two terms of four months each. Lectures were held in the evenings, six days a week. The students took notes and examined wet and dry specimens of muscle and bone. John prepared the specimens in the morning, demonstrated dissection and preservation during the day, and attended his brother's lectures at night. John was also put in charge of procuring the necessary number of cadavers. The bodies needed to be fresh, and they often needed to be of a particular gender (male or female), age (adult, child, or fetus), or condition (healthy or diseased). Some of these bodies were obtained from the gallows at Tyburn, probably by bribery but possibly by force, including two executed felons with severe gonorrhea. But to regularly supply the anatomy school with bodies, and to supply his own needs during his career, John turned necessarily to graverobbing. He was said to be a favorite of the local resurrectionists. One of his biographers states, "John Hunter would dissect more bodies, and therefore require more bodies stolen from graves, than any other anatomist of the eighteenth century" (Moore 2005). During the twelve years that he worked at William's school, John had — according to his own tally — been present at 2,000 human dissections. Moore (2005) concludes, "Given the sheer number of hours he spent poring over an endless stream of corpses, he had more opportunities to study the human interior than any other anatomist in Britain at the time."

John was usually discreet about the source of his cadavers, but revealed in one of his casebooks that he had obtained a "stout man" from St. George's burial ground in London in 1758. William warned his students at the start of each term to be mindful of upsetting the populace by keeping mum about the illegitimate sources of their cadavers: "Therefore it is to be hoped," he told them, "that you will be upon your guard; and, out of doors, speak with caution of what may be passing here, especially with respect to dead bodies" (Moore 2005). One body that John and William were particularly proud to have secured was that of a woman who had died very late in her pregnancy. Her body was fresh and, in William's words, "every part was examined in the most public manner" (Moore 2005). Though rare, it was not the only pregnant body they obtained. Between 1750 and 1754, the bodies of five pregnant and one recently post-partum woman were dissected and sketched at the school. The feat culminated in the later publication of William's monumental atlas, *The Anatomy of the Human Gravid Uterus*, although John was given no acknowledgment for his contributions.

1. Anatomists as Procurers of Cadavers (John Hunter)

The body of the "stout man" was used to demonstrate the muscles. The following year, John notes that he stripped the bones of an old woman who died in St. George's Hospital. His prowess, evidenced by shelves of expert preparations, enhanced the reputation of the school. He was named its instructor and demonstrator in 1749, only a year after he had arrived. He air-dried and varnished many of the teaching specimens, including bones, muscles, and organs. Others he preserved with solutions he developed himself and injected by syringe. He usually flushed out the blood vessels with water first. Lungs he inflated with air before introducing the embalming fluid, which was often colored with an artist's pigment. He prepared the lymphatic vessels by inflating and blowing mercury into them, and also prepared corrosion casts of blood vessels by injecting them with wax and submerging them in acid to remove the tissue around them. Most of John's preservations were appropriated by his brother without attribution, but the earliest specimen he was known to have retained as he started his own collection was a pair of nerves that led from the nose to the brain and which he pickled in wine.

In 1753, John began to take over some of his older brother's lectures, though he was never as poised at the podium (Moore 2005). In 1756, he became a house surgeon at St. George's hospital, which allowed him to apply his considerable knowledge of anatomy to living patients. But what the post also did was give him access to the patients who didn't survive. His casebooks of the time log numerous operations, but also detail the many autopsies of bodies in the hospital morgue awaiting burial — autopsies that were often requested by the families of the deceased. When William's school closed, John joined the army. With his focus on battlefield surgery and attending the wounded, he still took the time to add to his anatomical collection. As his biographer points out, "Army lifestyle had at least supplied the plentiful quantities of alcohol he needed for pickling his treasures" (Moore 2005). In 1763, John and William had the opportunity to unwrap an ancient Egyptian mummy at the house of a London physician. John had made a name for himself in medical circles, so when his colleagues learned that he would be conducting a postmortem examination, he could be sure of an audience (Moore 2005). One such crowd assembled to watch him perform an autopsy on a woman named Martha Rhodes, upon whom he had assisted in performing a caesarean section five hours earlier.

The Hunters had amassed a collection of some 15,000 anatomical specimens that were displayed in several rooms on the first floor of their school and residence. Many of these had been prepared by John, but when his older brother died in 1783, they passed by specific bequest to his student and nephew Matthew Baillie. The anatomical preparations — along with William's collection of books, coins, and paintings — reverted after thirty years to Glasgow University, where they are still conserved. Two years after William's death, John Hunter moved his family and the specimens he had been able to retain for himself to a new home in London. He continued to lecture about and demonstrate anatomy, in addition to attending surgical patients. The ground floor contained a roomy amphitheater equipped with semi-circular benches for his audience of students. At the center was a slate table which had wheels so that it could be positioned where the light was strongest. Both of the levels above the amphitheater were devoted to the anatomist's cherished museum.

The specimens were wet and dry, animal and human. The wet specimens were preserved in some five thousand flint glass jars that must have been custom-made, since they were not commercially available (Kobler 1988). In addition to those he had acquired during his dissections, he had purchased them from circuses, menageries, and auctions. His collection of infants included one born without a skull, another born with spina bifida, and a set of quintuplets who had each died during or shortly after birth. He had also acquired the double-skull of a six-year-old child and a woman's double-womb. About his monstrosities, John said, "From wrong construction of parts arises unnatural action, which by studying we may discover the natural actions" (Kobler 1988). Among the items from adults that he preserved were the penis of a man who had gonorrhea and the skull and bones of a long-term sufferer of syphilis. In 1770, he was pleased to add the sexual organs and vessels of an old army general named Robert Armiger, who likely died during sexual intercourse. And he had the deformed skeleton of a man with myositis ossificans, purchased for a steep price at an anatomical auction in 1783. He almost acquired the remains of Tobias Smollett upon his death in 1771, but although the novelist promised it to the anatomist in a letter, his widow

1. Anatomists as Procurers of Cadavers (John Hunter)

refused to release it (Moore 2005). Hunter did have specimens of named individuals in his collection in the form of diseased and damaged organs culled from the sanctioned autopsies of well-known and well-to-do British citizens. One autopsy from which a section of kidney was retained was that of his own father-in-law, retired surgeon Robert Home (Moore 2005).

There was a very notable living individual from whom John Hunter was driven to — and notorious for — deriving a skeleton for his collection. Charles Byrne was a well-known curiosity in London because of his great height, which was promoted at an exaggerated eight feet (although he certainly stood at least seven and a half feet tall). He had left his home in Ireland at the age of twenty-one in 1782 and found fame, but also succumbed to alcoholism. Within a year he was in very poor health and took the opportunity to extract a promise from his friends. In an attempt to thwart John Hunter and any other anatomist, he insisted that they seal his body in a lead coffin and sink it in the middle of the English Channel. But Hunter was determined to have the skeleton of the Irish Giant for his collection, so as soon as he heard that the young man had died in 1783, he sought out and bribed the undertaker charged with handling the remains. Although it cost him a considerable sum, John secured the body and paving stones were sunk instead. Byrne's body was delivered to London by cart under cover of darkness. John took possession of it, wrangling it into his basement laboratory before dawn. Abandoning his usual care in favor of haste, Hunter dismantled the body and boiled the pieces in a giant copper vat to separate the flesh from the bones. He was then able to articulate the giant skeleton. He kept his prize a secret for four years before showing it off to his friends, although the oversized feet of Byrne's skeleton hung down provocatively in the portrait by the renowned Sir Joshua Reynolds for which Hunter was convinced to sit in 1785.

John derided surgeons and anatomists who did not direct the dissection of their own bodies, even though this had included his own brother. He had intended his own anatomical collection to contain his own diseased heart and the Achilles tendon he had torn in 1766, both to be preserved in spirits, but they were not retained when his brother-in-law dissected the dissector's body. "In life, Hunter's heart had always been in his museum; in death, the museum would have been its most fitting resting place," writes one of his biographers (Moore 2005). In his will, John stated his intention that the collection be sold to the nation in its entirety so that the proceeds would support his family. Unfortunately, England was at war with France and could not afford even a meager purchase price. In 1799, the government finally agreed to pay fifteen thousand pounds for the 13,687 specimens. They were placed in the custody of what was soon renamed the Royal College of Surgeons in 1813. William Clift, who had taken care of the collection since his mentor Hunter's death, was named the collection's first curator, and it was insured against fire and loss. Unfortunately, Hunter's brother-in-law Sir Everard Home withheld, plagiarized from, and later burned the anatomist's original manuscripts, casebooks, correspondence, and the catalogs he had meticulously compiled to document the collection. Despite the lack of explanations to accompany the specimens, they drew thousands of visitors from around the world, including scientists and royals. To Hunter's original collection, Clift added more than 3,000 specimens, including the skeleton of the twenty-two inch tall "Sicilian Fairy" Caroline Crachiami, whose portrait John had previously obtained from her father. With acquisitions over the next two hundred years, the collection grew to more than 65,000 items. Unfortunately, the galleries were damaged by bombs during World War II. Of the original specimens prepared by the prodigious John Hunter, only 3,500 remain. But he would be happy to know that one of these is the skeleton of the Irish Giant.

Sir Astley Cooper (1768–1841) and His Boast

Sir Astley Cooper is considered one of the greatest surgeons and anatomists of his day. After studying under his uncle William Cooper at Guy's Hospital, he was apprenticed to anatomist Henry Cline at St. Thomas' Hospital in London. Cooper had become a skilled dissector under both of his teachers. He had become much sought after by the other anatomy students, not only because of his ready availability in the dissecting room, but because he coached them eagerly, knowing how much he learned from guiding them in their anatomical pursuits. He often noticed things that had been missed when he perused the cadavers in the process of being dissected. On many occasions, however, he preferred the opportunity to perform private dissections in Cline's home. He visited the anatomy department at the University of Edinburgh and attended lectures by Cline's mentor, Scottish surgeon John Hunter. In 1789, Cooper was appointed demonstrator in anatomy at St. Thomas', and in 1791 Cline allowed him to give lectures of his own. Cooper's class size swelled as his reputation increased. He went to the hospital to dissect before breakfast so that he would be prepared to demonstrate for, and lecture to, students in the afternoon. He was also responsible for embalming the subjects the students dissected.

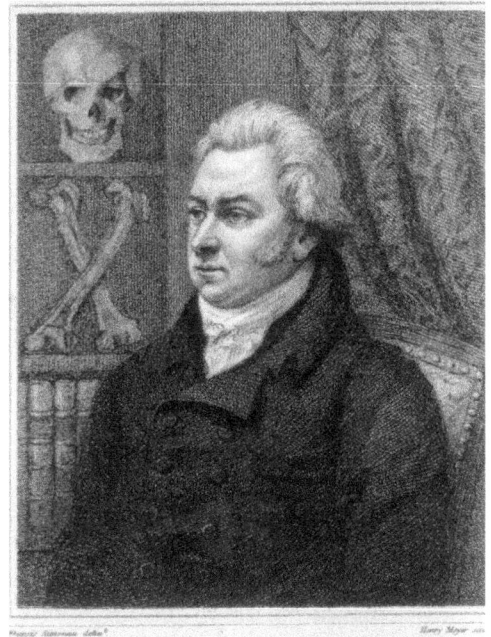

This portrait of English anatomist Sir Astley Cooper was published in 1819. Note the skull and crossbones behind his right shoulder (*courtesy National Library of Medicine*).

Cooper was appointed lecturer on anatomy to Surgeon's Hall in 1793, an honor for a man so young, but merited because he "had attained a degree of proficiency in anatomical knowledge, far beyond that possessed by any other of the pupils of his own standing in the hospital" (Cooper 1843). His duties were to dissect before members of his profession the criminals executed at the Old Bailey, and this he did until 1796. In 1805, he succeeded his uncle as surgeon at Guy's Hospital in London, in addition to maintaining a thriving private practice, and continuing to lecture in anatomy and surgery at St. Thomas' until 1825. His career had centered around teaching, dissection, and experimental surgery, the last of which benefited from the detailed case notes he was known to keep. To help quench his thirst for knowledge, Cooper paid men to secure and retrieve the bodies of patients up to one hundred miles away who had died during or following an operation so that he could learn, through a postmortem examination, what went wrong.

Cooper's occupation as a professor of anatomy and surgery necessitated dealing with bodysnatchers and, while his servant Charles often acted as go-between, Cooper knew these men so well that he was the best-supplied anatomist in London. His students were also compelled to steal bodies, which they did with full complicity of the professionals, as Cooper's biographer relates:

> The Hospital students would occasionally join the depredators in their nightly exploits, though not unfrequently obliged to pay for the danger which they thus incurred. They were, however, most frequently kept apart from the more important operations, being employed either in looking out or some such subordinate occupation: never as far as I know being allowed to engage themselves actively in the proceedings at the grave [Cooper 1843].

At times during Cooper's career at St. Thomas' Hospital, bodysnatchers deposited the corpses in hampers in the courtyard of his house. They would then be picked up by a porter who would transport them to the dissecting rooms. Arrangements were often made to secure bodies for the entire semester by paying a bodysnatcher an advance and an agreed-upon sum for each corpse to be supplied throughout the coming months. The body-snatchers, who had the upper hand, often extorted high prices from professors like Cooper by threatening to supply rival schools. As the number of both students and schools grew, it became even more difficult to obtain subjects for dissection, because the bodysnatchers had to plunder graveyards further and further away — and had to do so without attracting the attention of an increasingly wary populace.

One way to minimize the risk of exposure was to prepay a person for the use of his or her body after death. Cooper was not above making such offers, though they were sometimes rebuffed. One man who did accept his terms, William Williams, signed his name to a lengthy document characterized by legal language:

1. Anatomists as Procurers of Cadavers (Sir Astley Cooper)

> Sir, Being fully sensible of the uncertainty of this life, and of the mortality of my animated frame,—the tabernacle of my soul and of the living spirit that pervades it,—and my mind being impressed with the subject of the public benefit to be derived from anatomy, I beg, Sir, to communicate to you in writing, what in substance has already been submitted by personal communication to your notice, in regard to my body, graciously bestowed on me by my Maker, when the hereafter desertion of that body by its animated tenants of spirit and soul shall take place. If, Sir, in your lifetime, I die a bachelor or unmarried, within the Metropolis of Great Britain, called London, or within a convenient distance of the same, or whatever you may consider a convenient distance, I beg, with a view to the furtherance of useful knowledge in the science of anatomy, &c [Cooper 1843].

The gist of the text is that Williams' wife would have the right to cancel the bequest, but if he died without marrying, Cooper had the right to dissect or supervise the dissection of the man's remains.

Having suffered the risks and indignities—to their profession and to the dead—of the shortage of cadavers for years, Cooper supplied information to a House of Commons Committee that lobbied for a change in the law. The recommendation led to the enactment of the 1832 Anatomy Act. According to him, only 450 bodies were supplied to the Royal College of Surgeons each year, while the anatomy students in London numbered 700 annually. With at least four cadavers necessary to adequately train each student for a career in medicine, the city's actual need was at least 1,800. What they did not receive legitimately, the anatomists obtained illicitly. As he told the Committee, "[N]o dead person, however exalted, is safe from the activities of the resurrectionists: the law only enhances the price, and does not prevent the exhumation" (Cooper 1843). He found on a tour of France that cadavers were not as much in demand as was the observant instruction he was fortunate enough to have had—and to give, noting in his diary in 1834:

> Went with Mr Fisher to _____ and saw there the places for dissection, four *salles* of great magnitude, two of which had numerous bodies in them. The price is from 3 to 8 francs according as they have been opened or not. A large garden is attached, in which the students can walk, when they are fatigued. Yet it is badly managed, for the young men have no one to stand over them, and constantly instruct them in

the best mode of dissection, or to demonstrate what they lay bare. In short the young men form themselves into parties of three, one dissecting, one reading, and the other tracing [Cooper 1843].

Cooper's lectures, on the other hand, were found to be unsurpassed and his writings were considered to be of the highest quality by his contemporaries. Mindful of the difficulty anatomists outside the city had in obtaining bodies, he sent a well-selected cadaver to friend and colleague Joseph Swan at Lincoln County Hospital each Christmas in a large hamper labeled with instructions that it contained glass and should be handled with care. Cooper boasted of his ability to procure subjects for anatomy, stating before that committee of the House of Commons, "The law does not prevent our obtaining the body of an individual if we think proper; for there is no purpose, let his situation in life be what it may, whom, if I were disposed to dissect, I could not obtain" (Cooper 1843). He added that the law did not discourage such gruesome theft, it just inflated the prices of the cadavers. Before his own death, Cooper drew up specific directions for the dissection of his own body, and was afterward interred beneath Guy's Hospital.

2
Anatomists as Demonstrators and Educators

The Italian Renaissance signified not only the rebirth of art and culture, but the reemergence of the scholarly pursuit of anatomy. Surgeons, beginning with Mondino de Liuzzi in the fourteenth century, took up the scalpel and actively tested the prevailing animal-based second-century theories of Galen. Soon, dissections were being conducted publicly and privately, and were being observed by students, their professors, and interested observers. Where there were townspeople with questionable motives eager to get a glimpse of a rare female cadaver, there were also painters and sculptors attending to familiarize themselves with the underlying muscle structure of the figures they portrayed. The medical profession had already begun to distance itself from the specific identities of the cadavers they worked on, while it was later that the anatomists had to distance themselves from the bodysnatchers who supplied those bodies in the centuries that followed. Before the rivalry between the surgeons and physicians had sorted itself out, before the public preferred demonstrations on models that they could relate to their own health, and before the institutionalization of anatomy led eventually to the withdrawal of dissection from the public arena, heterogeneous crowds relished the fate of the cadaver with a medical — if morbid — interest. Guild members took pains to be included in group portraits of dissections by Rembrandt. And, most importantly, Vesalius demonstrated dynamically the secrets of the body, and the paramount necessity of seeing those secrets revealed with one's own eyes.

We know from fragmentary writings that human dissections were performed as early as the third century B.C. (Sawday 1995). Greek physician Herophilus and his contemporary Erasistratus (304–250 B.C.) taught

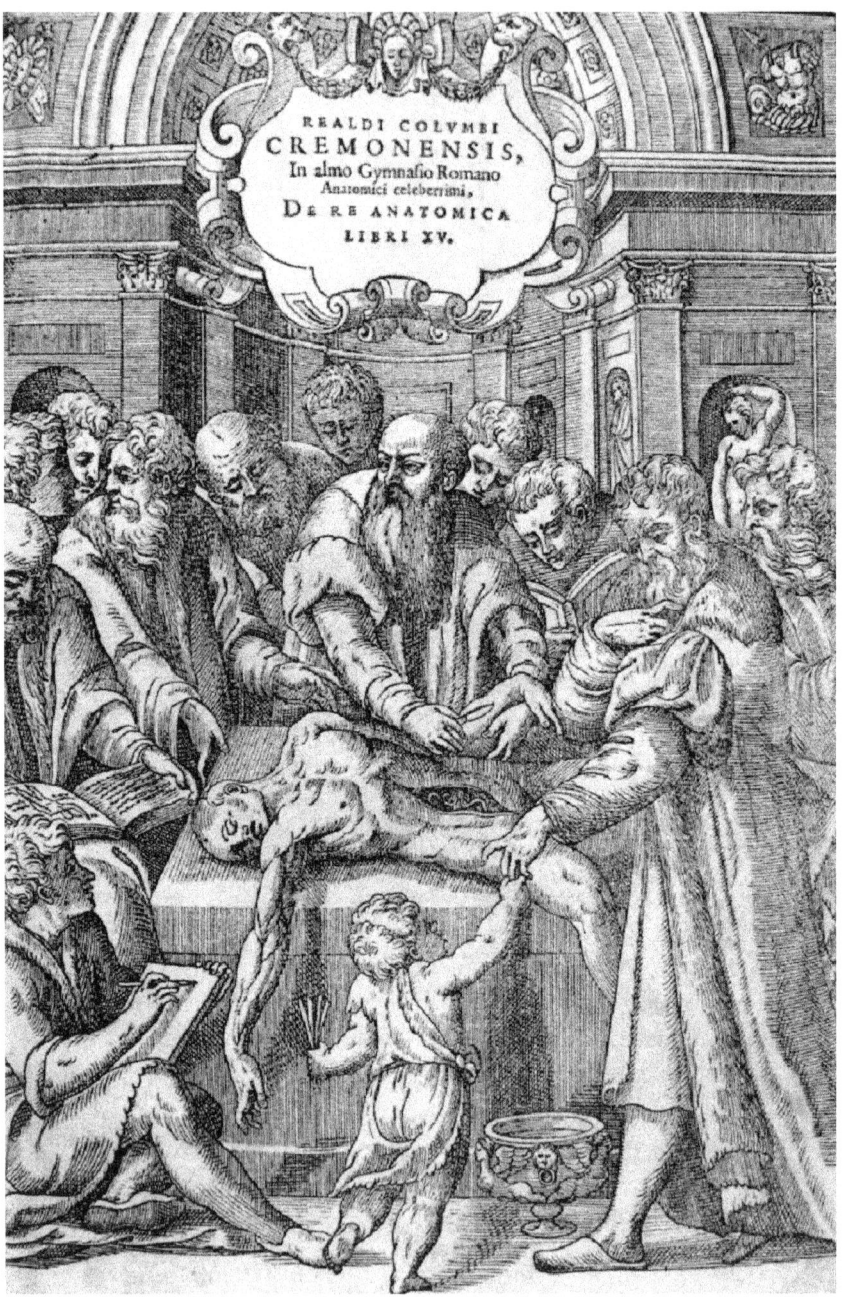

at the medical school in Alexandria, Egypt, and performed hundreds of dissections — often publicly — in one of the few places where dissecting human bodies wasn't banned. In fact, the academics associated with the Library of Alexandria were allowed during the reign of Ptolemy I (C. 367 B.C.–C. 283) to dissect the bodies of executed criminals. Herophilus is credited with introducing scientific method to medicine and making many anatomical discoveries, earning him the posterity of being considered the "father of human anatomy." But when the library was destroyed, the anatomical knowledge that had been gained was lost — and so, too, was the freedom to carry out further human dissections. They were. The field entered a fallow period that lasted some 1,500 years, dominated by the teachings of second-century Greek-born Roman physician Galen, who quoted Herophilus but by most accounts never replicated the earlier anatomist's direct observations from dissected human cadavers, a practice which was forbidden in ancient Rome. Instead, Galen extrapolated from his own dissections of animals, making few contributions of his own.

Anatomy was kept alive during the Middle Ages by Arabian physicians' translations of earlier Greek and Roman works. Human dissection was again taken up by a number of Arab physicians in the twelfth and thirteenth centuries, and practiced by surgeons in Christian Europe from the thirteenth century. Anatomy was regarded as a pagan science in Europe and a papal bull of 1299 prohibiting dissection is often cited as proof that the church disapproved of medical dissection, when in fact the instruction was meant to curb the practice of reducing the bodies of Christian crusaders to bones so that their remains could be transported home (Carlino 1999). The myth of medieval resistance to dissection is an old one. Opening the body was in fact common funerary practice from the early twelfth century, became tolerated in the fourteenth century, and didn't fall under suspicion until the mid-sixteenth century (Park

Opposite: Title page of Realdo Colombi's *Cremonensis*, published in Venice, 16th century. Anatomist Colombi had come to Padua to teach in place of Vesalius during his two-year stay in Switzerland to oversee the printing of *De humani corporis fabrica*. Vesalius and Colombi became bitter rivals, though Colombi's plans to collaborate with Michelangelo on a competing text never came to fruition. He published only one anatomy text, in which this image appears, in 1559 shortly before his death (*by permission of the Master and Fellows of St. John's College, Cambridge*).

1994). The stigma of public dissection was not about the opening of the body per se, but about the dramatic violation of family honor through publicly exposing the naked body, compromising its identifiability through mutilation, and forcing changes to the funeral ritual (Park 1994).

In the mid-thirteenth century, surgeons began to privilege their own observations over those of the classical authorities. One of these was William of Saliceto, whose anatomy text was topographical in nature and included structures he had seen and described. Although he was not an academician, Saliceto may have gained access to human cadavers through either forensic or funerary means. For families who could afford it, Saliceto may have prepared bodies for burial in more than one location — for instance, a person's heart at a shrine and the rest of the body at home, a tradition that necessitated dissection. (The association of dismemberment with the bodies of saints has been put forth to explain the general Italian tolerance of anatomy and dissection.) Or, at the request of church officials or city authorities, Saliceto may have performed autopsies to determine cause of death (Infusino et al. 1995). Bologna and other northern Italian cities appointed pool of doctors to testify in trials of suspected murder. A possible murder victim Azzolino degli Onesti was opened up at a judge's request in 1302 and found not to have died of poison; a woman named Ghisetta was autopsied in 1307, a procedure that concluded that she had died of internal bleeding from a wound that appeared superficially to have healed (Park 1994). Autopsies performed by doctors on their private patients became increasingly more common in the fifteenth century, as families concerned about hereditary disease requested it.

The technique of preeminent medieval French surgeon Guy de Chauliac (c. 1300–1368) is described below:

> Having laid the dead body on the table, [the anatomist] made four lessons on it. In the first the digestive members were treated since they decay the soonest. In the second the spiritual members, in the third, the animal organs and in the fourth the extremities were treated. And following the commentary ... there are nine things to see: that is to know the situation, the substance, the constitution, the member, the figure, the relation of connections, the actions and the uses and the diseases which affect them. Thus from anatomy the physician may gain

assistance and aid in the knowledge of diseases, in the prognosis and in the cure. We make anatomies also on bodies dried in the sun, or consumed in the earth, or immersed in running or boiling water. This shows us the anatomy at least of the bones, cartilages, joints, large nerves, tendons, and ligaments. By these two means we must teach anatomy on the bodies of men, apes, pigs, and many other animals, and not from pictures ... [Roberts and Tomlinson 1992].

Chauliac dissected in Montpellier every other year starting in 1340 (French 1999). He privileges actual dissection over book-learning, but may have extrapolated too much from his dissections of animals, as had Galen 1,000 years earlier.

By the end of the fifteenth century, the papal ban on dissection, which had never been very strictly observed at Padua and Bologna, had been lifted. Educational dissection was being carried out at the main universities of Europe: in Vienna since 1404, Prague since 1460, and Tubingen since 1485 (French 1999). Dissection became more than just a lesson to train a class of doctors, it became a spectacle attracting a wide range of scholars and artists. Artists who wanted to improve their modeling of the human figure looked beneath the skin of cadavers to see the underlying muscle structure. It was art that drove dissections which were *not* influenced by previous mistakes. The interest of artists and illustrators was also sustained by newly devel-

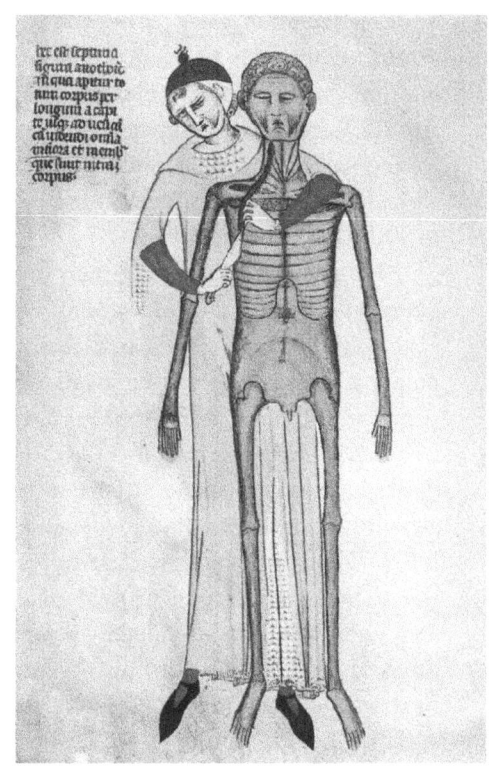

Dissection of a male cadaver, 14th century. This image was used to illustrate the anatomy text of Mondino de Liuzzi and Guido de Vigevano (*Wellcome Images*).

oped printing techniques that increased the availability of illustrated anatomy books. The subject of a 1450 altarpiece by Donatello entitled "The Miser's Heart," in which anatomists gaze into a cadaver's chest during a public dissection, suggests that he may have been the first Renaissance artist to perform a dissection (Lassek 1958). Among the first artist-dissectors to anatomize a human body so that he could accurately represent it in his art is said to be fifteenth-century Italian painter and sculptor Antonio del Pollaiuolo. Other Renaissance artists observed, carried out on their own, or served as demonstrators at dissections, often winning praise from later generations of anatomists. Scottish surgeon William Hunter said of Leonardo da Vinci, "When I consider what pains he has taken upon every part of the body, the superiority of his universal genius ... I am fully persuaded that Leonardo was the best Anatomist, at his time, in the world" (Hayes 2008). Both Michelangelo Buonarroti and da Vinci carried out human dissections in privacy, Michelangelo having gained access to bodies in the hospital awaiting burial and da Vinci secretly sketching anatomies in his notebooks until he was betrayed to and banned by the Pope.

Rather than conducting their own dissections, other artists simply attended the rare public dissections, which were sometimes held by guest anatomists. Paduan physician Galeazzo Santa Sofia, for instance, gave a public anatomy lesson using a cadaver when he visited Vienna in 1404 (Carlino 1999). According to Alessandro Benedetti, who taught in Padua from 1490 to 1495, anatomists liked to demonstrate their talents, particularly to well-known and important people who validated their work by allowing their names to be cited in anything the anatomists wrote (French 1999). Dissection was a privilege to perform and to observe. But in addition to being attended by learned men who chronicled the events, public anatomies were also attended by a nameless crowd that has left no trace. To paraphrase scholar Giovanna Ferrari (1987), these audience members were uneducated, unconcerned with the relationship between the political authorities and the university, unschooled in both Latin and anatomy, and possibly drawn by the promise of nudity — especially if admittance was free of charge.

In addition to living female bodies in the field of medicine, there was always a dearth of dead female bodies to dissect. The public anatomy of a woman was a rare event, and well-attended for reasons beyond the fact that it was instructional. When Italian physician Jacopo Berengario da Carpi anatomized a pregnant woman hanged in Bologna in the early sixteenth century (French 1999), it is likely that few members of the audience of five hundred university scholars and citizens were there to observe merely the embryonic membranes that were so carefully pointed out. For this reason, "he dismissed public dissections as useless displays, of interest only to tyros and curious townspeople. The true anatomist, he emphasized, worked in private, slowly and methodically, surrounded only by a handful of students" (Park 1994). Three hundred years later, an English crowd was smaller, but just as eager. The body of twenty-four-year-old Catherine Welsh was retrieved from the scaffold after she was hanged for the infanticide of her six-week-old son. Her body — one of only seven received by the Royal College of Surgeons between 1800 and 1832 — was dissected only perfunctorily. Instead, her head and shoulders were sketched by William Clift, who had been retained as the conservator of John Hunter's anatomical collections after the latter's death. The subject was then given over to Scottish anatomist Charles Bell, who ran a private school of anatomy and would have educated his students by dissecting the lactating breasts and vagina before opening the body to study the rest of the reproductive system (MacDonald 2005). Young upper class men had an excuse for any prurient interest, since they were encouraged to attend anatomy demonstrations and lectures whether or not they were taking up medicine (Nunn 2005).

The sixteenth century saw increased institutionalization of dissection. The first documented dissection in Rome took place in 1512, but Carlino (1999) explains that in that city at that time, anatomy remained of secondary concern. Public demonstrations often failed to be held, not because of a lack of cadavers, but because of a lack of personnel to dissect them. They were, however, performed regularly at Oxford beginning in 1549 and Cambridge beginning in 1565 (Sawday 1995). In the last quarter of the century, anatomists began to specialize and to conduct their own private "research anatomies" separate from the public anatomies held at the universities (French 1999). There was a continuing rivalry between the barber-surgeons, who had been granted the use of four bodies per year by King Henry VIII in 1540, and the university-trained members of the College of Physicians, who were allotted four bodies per year by Queen Elizabeth I twenty-five years later (Nunn 2005).

For centuries, physicians were held in much higher regard than surgeons. Physicians were the white-collar professors who treated the body from the inside. Barber-surgeons were the blue-collar operators who treated the body from the outside. The woodcuts of the time showed the hierarchy: the professor, holding his authoritative text, guided the proceedings from a lectern at the top of the theater, while the demonstrator, with rolled-up sleeves, applied his knife to expose the structure under discussion, the ostensor then pointing to it with a stick (French 1999). This arrangement began in the seventeenth century and meant that the anatomy theater had two foci: the dissecting table and the cathedra from which the professor propounded and defended his theses (Ferrari 1987). It was the hands-on demonstrating surgeon who — with the master and stewards of anatomy — was responsible for obtaining and preparing bodies for public and private dissections (Lassek 1958), and who spared professors from dealing directly with bodysnatchers (MacDonald 2005). The annual appointment was difficult to keep filled, but the position of lector could be, too. In Bologna, for instance, the reputation of the lector was at stake, so he was difficult to recruit even when given a full stipend. During the short but demanding anatomy course, the lector had to answer all questions put to him without prior warning by lectors from other disciplines. As an incentive, medals were given to the debaters to encourage them, and anatomy professors who distinguished themselves received special acknowledgment and gained an uncommon degree of prestige (Ferrari 1987).

One man who had a good reputation as a lecturer was seventeenth-century English physician William Harvey, best known as the first person to correctly describe the circulation of the blood in the human body. Harvey held public dissections during the winter months at London's Barber Surgeons Hall. Using the approach he had learned at Padua, Harvey discussed the causes, functions, and purposes of anatomical structures rather than simply identifying them, and is said to have remarked that he never conducted a dissection in which he did not make some new discovery (Wilson 1987). His lecture notes, intended for his own use during dissections, were published more than two hundred years after his death and, according to the introduction, "give a picture of him as no carefully prepared work could, delivering his lectures with a body dissected on the table before him, and a demonstrator who lifted up or exposed this part or that, at his bidding. There can be no doubt that the lectures interested their audience. Harvey never tries to appear learned, his whole aim seems to be to make the subject clear; there is no affectation, every remark has the stamp of his own original, thoughtful, observing mind" (Royal College 1886). Harvey's remarks seem deliberately designed to elicit laughter during his presentation, which would have caused his audience to look at a dissector in a new way — less an authority acting on the cadaver, which is momentarily forgotten, than an actor seeking to entertain and becoming as much an object of attention as the body on the table (Wilson 1987). The guidance that the anatomist laid out for his public lectures included demonstrating the features of the particular body on the table, omitting the discussion of anything that could as easily be learned without a cadaver present, dissecting as much as possible before the audience, and *avoiding praising or dispraising other anatomists*. Despite this last rule, these dissections disparaged the surgeons in his audience in favor of the socially and professionally preferred physicians. The surgeons, while intended to be the primary beneficiaries of the lectures, were ignorant of both anatomy and Latin, the language in which the dissections were conducted. So it is thought that Harvey's public anatomy demonstrations were more of a political than a medical event, intended not to raise the profile of the surgeons but rather to continue to exert control over them (Wilson 1987).

The rivalry between the physicians and the surgeons extended to anatomical dissection long after the social position of the dissectors had begun to improve in the fifteenth century (Ferrari 1987). Although the barber-surgeons had the upper hand because they had access to a legal allotment of bodies, they often had to call in physicians to educate their members during quarterly dissections (Nunn 2005). In late seventeenth-century Edinburgh, the town council gave the Royal College of Surgeons permission to dissect the bodies of foundlings, suicides, executed criminals, and those who died in workhouses. This privilege was predicated on erecting a permanent anatomical theater and holding an annual public dissection. As a means of "preventing extraneous hands in meddling in their matters" (Gairdner 1860), the surgeons appointed one of their own, Robert Elliot, as public dissector and authorized a salary of fifteen pounds per year for the next twelve years (Lassek 1958). But in the late eighteenth century, after the status of the surgeons had been raised, the competing groups began to cooperate. Academics curried favor by gifting the bodies that had been dissected to surgeons studying or working at London's charitable hospitals. This allowed the physicians to maintain close relationships with powerful surgeons, and in return procured from the surgeons reports that added to the body of anatomical and surgical knowledge (MacDonald 2005).

Despite the sharing, the lack of bodies to dissect meant that the few cadavers that were made available were shared among many anatomists for use in instructing their students. The subjects of dissection in European anatomy schools were executed prisoners, and often a gap of two or three years went by before the next body became available. At some schools, a student may see only a single dissection during his entire medical career. The statutes at the University of Bologna stipulated that students could attend only two male and one female anatomies in the entire course of their studies (Ferrari 1987). When the study of anatomy was offered at the University of Paris after the fourteenth century, the dissection of a hanged criminal between three and five times per year was a week-long public event. But in France, there was less stigma associated with dissection and a willingness to donate one's body, as French bishop St. Francis de Sales hoped to do: "I wish really for only one thing, that when I have expired, you shall deliver my body over to the doctors to perform the anatomy of it; it will be a relief to me to know that at least I shall serve the public in some way being dead, since I have been of no service during my life" (Ferrari 1987). In the nineteenth century, Paris was distinguished for its method of instruction in which each student was afforded a corpse for dissection. But in England, Scotland, and the rest of Europe, dissection was carried out on one body at a time, with an audience of students who did not actively participate. In fact, the instructor usually did not get his hands dirty — he lectured, while a demonstrator opened and dissected the cadaver.

Not all teachers of anatomy were associated with universities. From the eighteenth century, medical education was transacted on a private basis and some anatomists conducted lectures from their homes. Scottish surgeon William Hunter placed an advertisement to attract students to his home in 1746:

> On Monday, the 13th of October, at 5 in the evening will begin a course of anatomical lectures to which will be added the operations of surgery with the application of bandages, by William Hunter, surgeon. Gentlemen may have the opportunity of learning the art of dissection during the whole winter season in the same manner as at Paris...

Such teachers relied on the black market in corpses, either by patronizing the bodysnatchers or by becoming graverobbers themselves, and sometimes their reputations suffered. Scottish physician Andrew Moir of Aberdeen was widely disliked, not only because he taught in his own anatomy theater in direct competition with Marischal College (later the University of Aberdeen), but for the bodysnatching he was known to do — and to compel his students to do. The anger of the locals spilled over in 1831 and Moir's "Burkin' Hoose," as it was known, was ransacked and burned to the ground.

William Cheselden was called before his colleagues at the Barber Surgeons Company to explain why he had been dissecting the bodies of executed criminals for three years in his home and teaching from them without consent. The guild was entitled to the bodies of four executed criminals per year (later substituted with stillbirths and suicides) and so these subjects should have been publicly anatomized in Surgeon's Hall. Because he was popular, Cheselden was fined but forgiven, and granted permission to conduct regular lectures at his home and at St. Thomas's Hospital. This began a gradual relaxation of standards which encouraged the establishment of private anatomy schools, but also led to an additional demand for bodies which was filled by bodysnatchers (Lassek 1958). Private dissections were also controlled and legitimized by the universities when it was realized that students needed more practical experience than could be gained at public dissections. Some physicians already conducted private dissections, so students were prompted to form smaller anatomy seminars for the same purpose (Carlino 1999). In Van Dieman's Land in the nineteenth century, anatomies following execution were carried out in hospital dissecting rooms. Colonial surgeon James Scott invited medical men and men of his acquaintance, including artists and members of the press, to these events. But he strongly resisted — and was admonished for — attempts by private instructors to bring their pupils (MacDonald 2005).

While the sources of corpses for dissection were disputed in the nineteenth century, there were few voices raised to question the necessity of dissection itself and to suggest that more could be learned by observing the course of a fatal illness than examining the structure afterward (Richardson 1987). However, by then the public profile of anatomy had undergone a number of changes that eventually led to the discontinuation of the public dissection. Enthusiasm for anatomy's theatrical aspects waned as scholars questioned the scientific and educational value of such events. The professional training of doctors and surgeons was valued more highly than their oratorical skills or the perpetuation of prestigious traditions (Ferrari 1987). It was no longer the mark of a good anatomist to dissect as many bodies as possible to know what was normal so that he could convey the information as economically as possible in a single public dissection (French 1999). On the part of the public and the professionals, dissection had grown to become an embarrassment after the mid-eighteenth century. Physicians found it crude and no longer considered it an end in itself, but a stepping stone to other disciplines that had branched off, like pathology (Sappol 2002). Far from its early connection with the barber-surgeons, anatomy had become an essential core in the medical curriculum and the credentialing process, and surgery had become respectable. Medical men used their anatomical training to displace midwives, who were barred from practicing dissection until the 1840s, when they began to enter the medical profession (Sappol 2002).

There was both fascination with and disgust for dissection in the modern sensibility. The surgeons were still associated with the illicit and morally dubious means of obtaining bodies by haggling for them at the gallows or sanctioning their being dug up from their graves, and still had not achieved the status of physicians, who avoided coming into contact with the dead. The subjects of dissection continued to be considered unclean, disgusting things. And although interest in the secrets of the body had long ago overcome the taboos about scrutinizing it, at some point the corpse ceased to be the star of the show. Laypeople became disgusted by anatomy in favor of what was now called "physiology" and what it could teach them about their own health. Public exhibitions substituted artistic waxworks and other models for authentic bodies, for instance the ticketed anatomy lectures offered in 1762 by Philadelphia by Professor William Shippen, Jr., who demonstrated on models as well as cadavers. The attitude toward dead bodies had completely changed and repugnance toward everything associated with death had arisen. Public dissections once thought festive were now considered macabre and barbaric. Having outlived their educational, promotional, and scientific purposes, they no longer had reason to exist, not even as spectacle (Ferrari 1987).

One convention of contemporary educational dissection is to protect the identity of the deceased, but this safeguard has roots that go back centuries. A 1442 decree in Bologna mandated that bodies be obtained from at least thirty miles outside the city, so that the dissection could be carried out without the threat of a disturbance. The two bodies dissected annually in Padua and Pisa were never doctors, students, or local residents (Carlino 1999). In fact, it was routine throughout much of Europe to bring in the body from a nearby town when holding a public dissection and to avoid announcing the name of the subject out of respect for family—although the reason for the person's criminal conviction was stated so that the moral lesson was made explicit (van Dijck 2005). In addition to preventing any objections to the dissection by friends and relations, anonymity made the body representative rather than specific so that it could be used to obtain and demonstrate general knowledge. In an even larger sense, forestalling any identification of the cadaver as person was a triumph of scientific reason, with the aim of minimizing and eventually erasing the presence of the corpse—and perhaps even the dissector—from the iconography of anatomy (Sappol 2002).

Anatomists had also gotten past the religious taboos about dissection through their mediation of the cadaver, long considered unclean and unable to be resurrected after death. Once Christian doctrine clarified that mutilation of the body didn't preclude its being made whole again, dissectors had only to battle the substantial amount of superstition about the dead. One way they did this was to draw analogies between the hand of the cadaver and the hand of the dissector, emphasizing their function and the spiritual authority that inhabits both—God's hand (Rowe 1997).

The hand became the prominent vehicle for integrating sacred mystery with corporeal mechanism and was used to illustrate God's design (Carlino 1999). The history of anatomy was a battle between reason and superstition, and physicians and surgeons now defined themselves and their knowledge of the body in opposition to magic, charms, and powers (Sappol 2002), but not necessarily as a godless endeavor.

In nineteenth-century Europe, the progress of anatomy was hampered by regulations which shaped the organization of the anatomy lesson and the legal procedures by which the universities had access to cadavers (Carlino 1999). In the U.S., the dissecting tables in the medical schools were still supplied in large part by bodysnatchers (discussed below), because the anatomy laws did not keep up with the need. At the same time, the surgery required on the casualties of the Civil War by the many medical men and students who had enlisted intensified the anatomization of American medicine (Sappol 2002). Legislation began to address the need for accessible cadavers. By the early twentieth century, only a few American states with medical schools had not yet passed laws permitting them to appropriate the bodies of the indigent for dissection. When the bodysnatching scandals disappeared from the headlines, anatomical dissection was made invisible, as it remains today (Sappol 2002). The anatomy demonstration was still done, but it was done behind closed doors.

It wasn't until the late twentieth century — with the advent and improvement of CT and MRI technologies and 3D computer imaging — that the relevance of the actual physical dissection of a corpse has been debated. And the consensus seems to be that direct dissection of a cadaver has an educational value that cannot be entirely supplanted by the alternative methods for learning anatomy. To date, successful completion of Gross Anatomy I remains mandatory for medical students, and many of them mark the course as a turning point. Not only is it the first opportunity to develop the clinical detachment necessary for a medical career, it is a shared experience that marks the entry into the medical fraternity — a group that is cloaked both literally and figuratively. The gathering of the white-frocked doctors-to-be around a dissected cadaver in the photographs reproduced in the book *Dissection*, is called by authors John Harley Warner and James M. Edmonson "collaborative learning" and a "communal rite of passage."

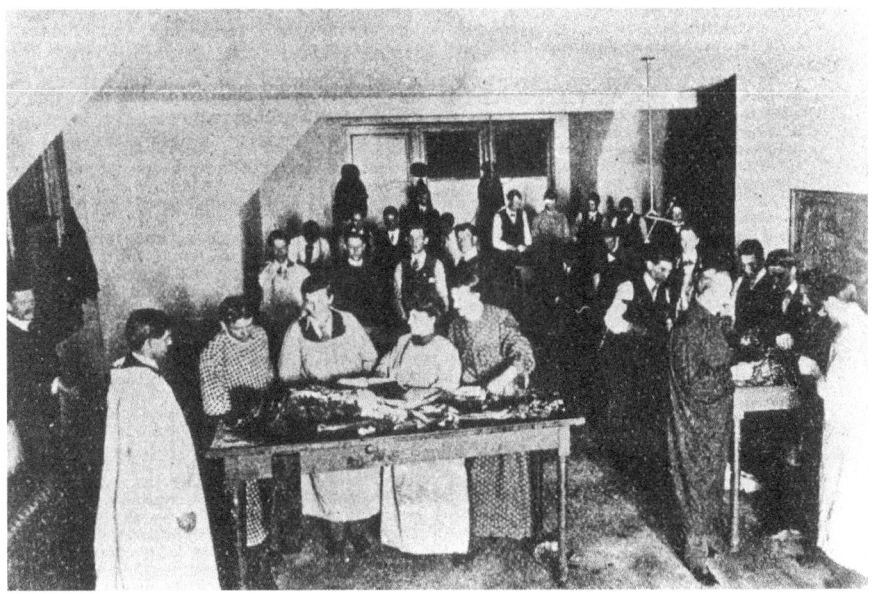

This photograph of the dissecting room at Chattanooga Medical College from the 1903-1904 school year shows students, some of them in full-length smocks, at work dissecting cadavers in the anatomy classroom of Professor Ellis and Dr. Woolford (*courtesy National Library of Medicine*).

In *Body of Work*, Montross (2007) describes her feelings as the dissection of her team's cadaver in her gross anatomy class progresses over the course of the semester. One of the first things she notices is how much work is involved in dismantling a human corpse, and notes the toll on her own body in both physical and emotional ways. "The force necessary in the dissections feels barbarous, and I am still fascinated by what is revealed but hate the push and tug necessary for revelation," she records in her journal. Regarding the emotional component, Montross explains that is made easier by working with others in the anatomy lab: "In order to dissect, we detach from what we are doing, and that detachment is easier to accomplish in a crowd." Even as the cutting gets easier, all through the semester she is struck by the ways in which the cadavers remind the students that they were once as alive as their dissectors:

> My sense of the humanity of our cadavers is evasive and shifting. One of the strangest things about dissecting a human body is the difference

between a human body and a human being — in some ways readily identifiable and in others barely perceptible. Everything tangible that is human is present in our cadavers. Their dead body parts are structurally identical to our living ones. Our cadavers are undeniably human.

Montross writes after the experience, "Yet there is no shortage of mystery in the body for me today, even after having cut it apart and held its wildly various shapes and tissues in my hands." In the end, even participatory dissection may not satisfy legitimate (or merely morbid) curiosity.

To have merit as an instructive technique, the process of dissection must be shared with others. Whether this means observing a dissection from the audience or cutting apart a corpse while standing shoulder to shoulder with fellow students, "public" dissection does impart knowledge. It is the context in which the body is breached that determines if a dissection is merely educational or crosses the line into entertainment — and whether this is acceptable or transgressive.

Mondino de Liuzzi (C. 1270–1326) and His History

Mondino de Liuzzi was born into prominent medical family in Florence in the thirteenth century. He studied at the University of Bologna and after graduating took a position there in the early fourteenth century as a public lecturer in practical medicine and surgery. In 1315, Mondino became the first post–Alexandrian to completely dissect a human body. He performed this dissection, which had been sanctioned by the pope, in the presence of students and spectators. The subjects were two executed prisoners (Carlino 1999), both of them female, and it has been suggested (Wilson 1987) that the anatomist was probably allowed to choose their method of execution. Although the dissection would have been ritualized and mechanical — with Mondino reading aloud from an anatomy text, a demonstrator doing the cutting, and an ostensor pointing to the relevant body parts with a wand — this event was the turning point in the revival of human anatomy.

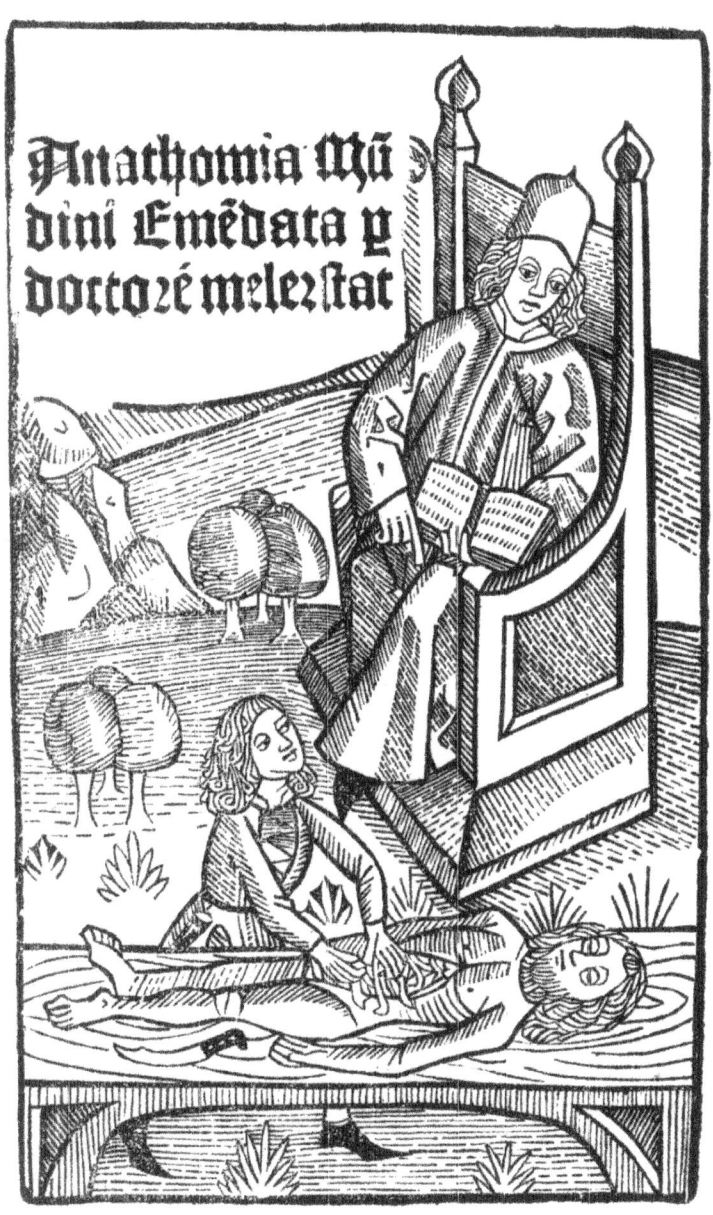

This illustration from a German edition of Mondino de Liuzzi's classic anatomy text *Anatomia corporis humani,* published circa 1493, shows a dissection being conducted in the open air under the direction of a professor who consults a text from his position of prominence in an elevated throne-like chair (*Yale University, Harvey Cushing/John Hay Whitney Medical Library*).

Mondino incorporated a systematic study of anatomy and dissection into the medical curriculum. His methods included drying the cadaver in the sun rather than hurriedly dissecting it as it decayed. He subscribed to the idea that the body consisted of three parts and that its dissection should begin with the basest and most inferior. The demonstration should begin with the "inferior ventricle" or abdomen, the organs of which were the most confused and least noble. Second, the anatomist should dissect the "middle ventricle" or thorax, which contained the more spiritual organs like the heart and lungs. Lastly, the "superior ventricle" or skull, which contained the higher organized structures, should be opened. Mondino prescribed one set of specific methods for the dissection of simple body parts like bones, muscles, and blood vessels, and another set of instructions for demonstrating complex structures like eyes and ears.

Only a year after his first public dissection, Mondino incorporated his methods into a work considered to be not only the first anatomical textbook, but the first modern dissection manual. *Anathomia corporis humani* had been printed in dozens of editions by the fifteenth century and was the most widely used anatomical text through the sixteenth century. Not only did it include the technical steps involved in the dissection of the human cadaver, it laid out the reason behind the way these steps were organized. In his *Anathomia*, Mondino first asserts that humans are superior to all other creatures because they can reason, use tools, and stand upright. He then explains how to access the various organs by means of specific incisions and describes many of them, including the stomach and spleen, in great detail.

Mondino bases *Anathomia* on twelfth-, thirteenth-, and fourteenth-century translations of the writings of Greek and Islamic scholars (Infusino et al. 1995). In doing so, he incorporates a number of fallacies, often in an attempt to reconcile the teachings of Galen and Aristotle. Some of his descriptions, such as the Aristotelian notion that the heart has three chambers, were inaccurate. And although he correctly stated that the uterus increased in size during menstruation and pregnancy, he perpetuated the notion that the organ was horned and had seven cells. And this is despite the accepted claim that he dissected the bodies of two women before an audience in 1315. Mondino does introduce some new and correct observations, and he does stress the experience gained by his own direct observations during dissection. So although his work was not entirely accurate, Mondino was considered a master, and the adoption of his textbook was mandated in many medical schools, making him particularly influential among academics during the centuries leading up to Vesalius.

Andreas Vesalius (1514–1564) and His Modernity

Revolutionary Belgian anatomist Andreas Vesalius (1514–1564) received his medical degree in Padua and was immediately appointed there as an instructor. It was through his human dissections that Vesalius demonstrated the flaws of second-century Greek physician Galen, whose animal-based theories had until then been universally accepted. Vesalius carried out the demonstrations himself during his lectures, and encouraged his students to dissect. Notes taken by one of his pupils during his first dissection are still preserved:

> The anatomy of our subject was arranged in the place ... they use to elect the Rector medicorum: a table on which the subject is laid, was conveniently and well installed with four steps of benches in a circle, so that nearly 200 persons could see the anatomy. However, nobody was allowed to enter before the anatomists, and after them, those who had paid 20 sol. More than 130 students were present and D. Curtius, Eregus, and many other doctors, followers of Curtius. At last, D. Andreas Vesalius arrived, and many candles were lighted, so that all should see, etc. ... And there was the body, cut up and prepared beforehand, already shaved, washed and cleaned. He began with the outer skin ... [Roberts and Tomlinson 1992].

In addition to his teaching duties at Padua, Vesalius was honored with an invitation to conduct two public dissections a year at the University of Bologna, probably in the years 1539 and 1540. A special wooden building, which he described as "elegant," was erected for the event. A large and select gathering was present to witness the first demonstration, and Vesalius handled it in a grandiose fashion. On that occasion, three bodies were turned over for dissection. At the second dissection, he anatomized the bodies of a human and an ape, later presenting their skeletons to the faculty. At a subsequent lecture, Vesalius promised his audience — which consisted mainly of students, with an additional fifty or so doctors and learned people present — that they would have a fresh subject the next day because a man was due to be hanged and "indeed this cadaver is now dry and wrinkled" (Ferrari 1987).

Vesalius was known to snatch bodies and to rob the gibbet to supply adequate anatomical material for his demonstrations. He encouraged his students, either by word of mouth or through anecdotes in his writings, to do the same. If they were to learn anatomy directly, as he strongly advocated, they had to go to the source. At the time, that meant the gallows and the cemetery, so Vesalius had no shame about this. He passed his determination on to the practitioners at his public dissections, which were often followed by waves of bodysnatching. Unlike the respect carefully shown to today's cadavers, Vesalius showed a lack of respect toward the bodies he stole from their resting places, and a particularly candid amusement about snatching female corpses. He and his students forged keys, rifled tombs and gibbets, and violated ossuaries in nighttime escapades. He brags about obtaining the body of the mistress of a monk, whose skin was flayed so that she would not be recognized (Park 1994).

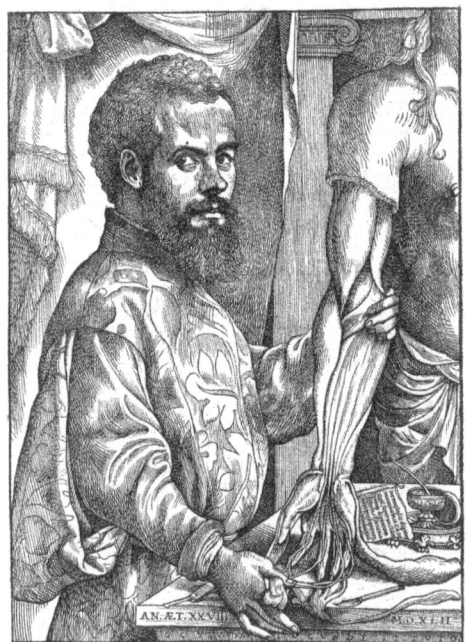

In this portrait from his 1543 text *De humani corporis fabrica*, anatomist Andreas Vesalius is shown demonstrating the musculature of the arm (*courtesy National Library of Medicine*).

Vesalius's concern was

instruction. When the students in his audience were boisterous, he sent them all outside and let them return only in small groups to see prepared dissections. He was also known to make quick charcoal sketches during dissections to show the shape and relationship of the parts as they were progressively destroyed (French 1999). And although the book was not intended to substitute for actual dissection, Vesalius published his classic seven-volume text *De humani corporis fabrica [On the Fabric of the Human Body]*. The work is considered one of the greatest medical books ever written, significant because it was the first time anatomy had been based on objective observation, accurate recording and presentation of data, and the pursuit of concepts to their logical conclusions (Malomo et al. 2006). *Fabrica* did extend medical knowledge to others in the absence of bodies to examine. But Klestinec (2006) argues that the famous illustration on its title page speaks to print technology, showing that dissec-

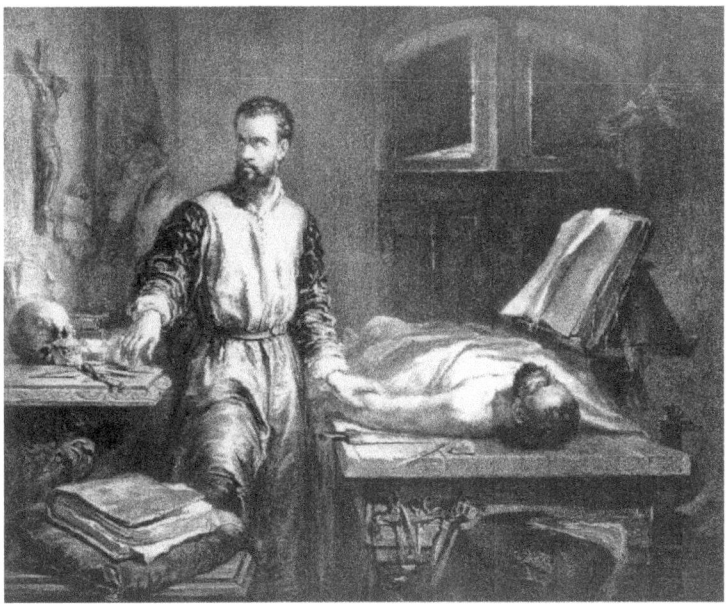

Andreas Vesalius in Padua, 16th century. The man who revolutionized anatomy with his "hands-on" approach stands between tables gazing at a crucifix. The table on the left holds a skull and his instruments. On the right is a cadaver, behind which stands an anatomical folio. The image is after a 19th-century painting by E.J.C. Hamman (*Wellcome Images*).

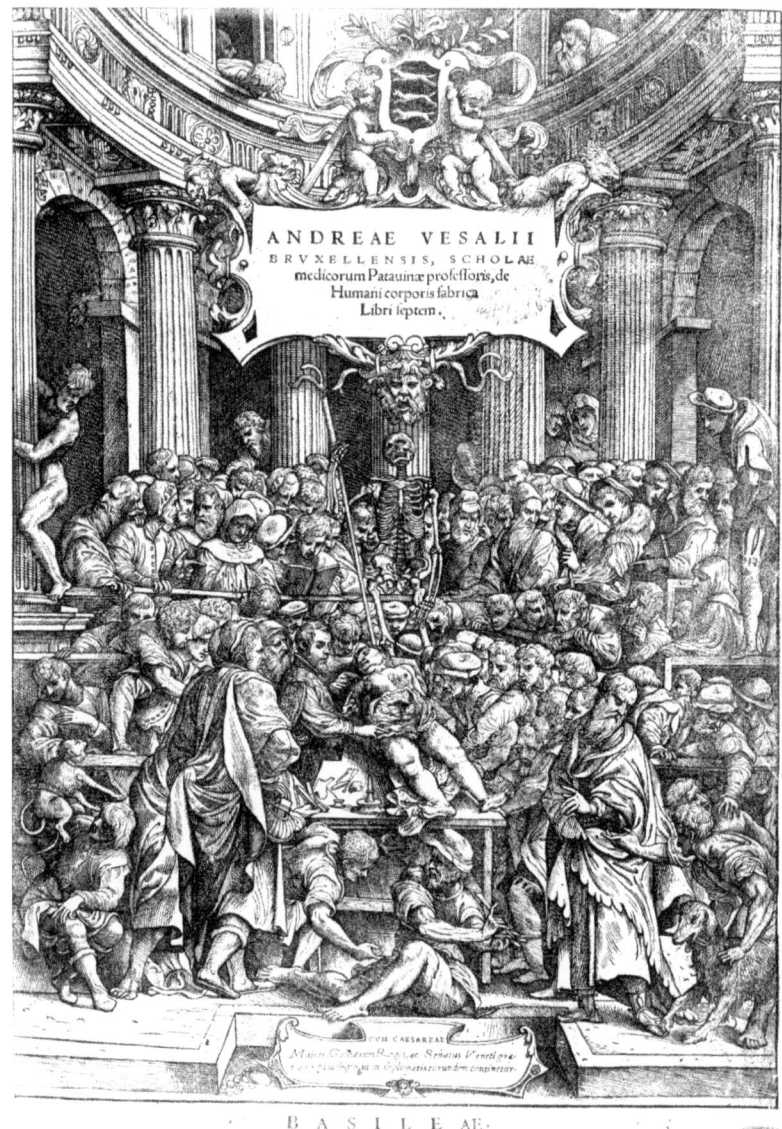

This illustration on the title page of Vesalius's 1543 textbook *De humani corporis fabrica [On the Fabric of the Human Body]* depicts a busy anatomy theatre with Vesalius at the center conducting his own dissection and trusting his own hands rather than relying on those of the demonstrator (*courtesy National Library of Medicine*).

2. Anatomists as Demonstrators and Educators (Andreas Vesalius)

tion is an intimate ritual within a tightly-knit medical community and reconciling the transmission of knowledge by the manual art of dissection with the distanced readership of the book.

Vesalius criticized the public anatomy lesson because the physicians read descriptions from outdated textbooks and the barber-surgeons who actually did the dissections during the lecture were unaccustomed to public speaking, so the whole thing was ruined as a demonstration (Carlino 1999). He expressed his disapproval of the ineffective the traditional dissection in the preface to his most famous book:

> These latter [the lectors] are perched up aloft in a pulpit like jackdaws, and with a notable air of disdain they drone out information about facts they have never approached at first hand, but which they merely commit to memory from the books of others, or of which they have descriptions before their eyes; the former [the dissectors] are so ignorant of languages that they are unable to explain their dissections to the onlookers and botch what ought to be exhibited in accordance with the instruction of the physician, who never applies his hand to the dissection, and contemptuously steers the ship out of the manual. Thus everything is wrongly taught, days are wasted in absurd questions, and in the confusion less is offered to the onlooker than a butcher in his stall could teach a doctor [Downs 2004].

Vesalius espoused multi-tasking: the person doing the dissection should not only be familiar with the classic anatomical texts and their inconsistencies with the actual cadaver, but he should also be able to explain and demonstrate these at the same time. The lector and dissector should be a single individual.

The image in *Fabrica* shows a crowd gathered around the anatomist and has been seen as illustrative of Vesalius' human-centered approach and an actual public dissection. As influential as it was, much of the imagery was idealized and symbolic. As it was in Padua and Bologna, the anatomical theater is depicted as a temporary structure erected whenever a public anatomy was held. The crowd consists of students, professors, clerics, physicians, and commoners who can be distinguished by their dress and attitudes. In the right foreground, in classical dress, is a figure convincingly thought to be Galen, and the monkey on the left refers to his dissection of animals and the\ mistaken assumption that their interiors are identical to humans. The unskilled barber-surgeons are relegated to the foot of the dissecting table, where they sharpen the knives. Depiction of the dissection table itself is completely innovative and overthrows the relationship between theory and practice. Upsetting the usual hierarchy, it is the teacher himself who dissects the cadaver, with his right hand thrust into the body and his left hand raised as if to emphasize the words that accompany the demonstration. The equal importance of written and practical knowledge is underlined by the inclusion of an inkwell, a pen, and a sheet of paper on the table next to the surgical instruments, and the figure to the right who both holds a book and points toward the dissecting table (Carlino 1999).

Although many of the elements of the illustration reflect features of the actual practice, they generally do so in exaggerated form. This includes the subject of the dissection, who is vertically oriented in the image and thus participatory rather than inert. The spectators themselves — all potential subjects of dissection — form spectacles both for one another and for the outside observer. The central performance is both of and by anatomist and cadaver (Wilson 1987). The crowd gathering around the table probably accurately depicts the direct involvement that Vesalius encouraged in his students. But by performing the dual roles of lecturer and dissector, Vesalius was the star of the show (Nunn 2005). He is universally reported to have kept his audience spellbound and his anatomy demonstrations were conducted with ceremony, decorum, and discipline (Wilson 1987). Nevertheless, it was several more decades before the university progressed to a model in which lector and dissector were one and the same (Carlino 1999). Vesalius's method was revolutionary. He knew it and influenced not only his contemporaries, but all anatomists who followed.

John Bell (1763–1820) and His Illustrations

Like William Hunter, John Bell was a distinguished Scottish anatomist, surgeon, and lecturer. He studied in his native Edinburgh under teachers including Alexander Monro secundus. It was written of him (Walls 1964) that he was as fortunate in his teachers as his students were to be in him. He described his studies in one of his books:

> In Dr. Monro's class, unless there be a fortunate succession of bloody murders, not three subjects are dissected in the year. On the remains of a subject fished up from the bottom of a tub of spirits are demonstrated those delicate nerves which are to be avoided or divided in our operations; and these are demonstrated once at the distance of 100 feet!— nerves and arteries which the surgeon has to dissect, at the peril of his patient's life [Walls 1964].

Despite the shortcomings that the lack of cadavers posed, John absorbed his lessons and was able to pass them on. After his studies, he drew large crowds to his demonstrations at the anatomical theater in Surgeons' Square. There he was, again like Hunter, assisted by his younger brother. Charles Bell had already distinguished himself as a student at the University of Edinburgh, by illustrating and publishing *A System of Dissection Explaining the Anatomy of the Human Body*. They both became members of the College of Surgeons of Edinburgh, and Charles operated with success at the Royal Infirmary, while John built up a successful private surgical practice and by 1799 he discontinued conducting well-attended private anatomy lessons in its favor. His reputation extended far beyond Edinburgh, and he operated at the top of his profession for more than twenty years.

In an unfortunate turn of events, attributed to the jealousy of their colleagues toward their popularity and their outspokenness about the pain caused by surgical incompetence, the Bells had been banned — along with the rest its junior members — by the College of Surgeons from operating in its infirmary. Even though John fought the decision strenuously and Charles offered to pay for the privilege of being "allowed to stand by the bodies when dissected in the theatre of the infirmary, and to make notes and drawings of the diseased appearances," the decision stood. They were forced to discontinue anatomizing, sketching, and preserving specimens from the bodies of patients who died in the infirmary. In 1802 Charles moved, with the museum he had assembled, to London where he gave anatomical lectures to painters, conducted private dissections, and grew his surgical practice. John's activities took him to Europe and he later died in Italy. Charles returned to the University of Edinburgh, where he accepted the chair of surgery and a knighthood by the British crown.

Both brothers had published numerous well-received surgical and anatomical textbooks. The books John Bell wrote, including *Anatomy of the Human Body* with which he shared credit with his brother, were known for being thorough (reviewing historical and outlining contemporary treatment) and clear (offering clinical examples). Wary of trusting the illustration of his books to artists, and like his brother having as talented a hand with a pen as with a scalpel, he had created the anatomical plates for them himself. He believed that artists and anatomists often worked at cross purposes, with illustrators aiming for aesthetic appeal and dissectors attempting to achieve accurate and useful representation. Many of his engravings are now considered landmarks in the field. In the preface to his *Engravings of the Bones, Muscles and Joints*, Bell wrote:

> Dissection is the first and last business of the student; and when drawings are made for his use, the body should be laid out as he is to order it in dissection; the belly should be displayed as he can display it in his subjects; an arm should be so drawn, that, when he dissects the arm of the subject, it may fall naturally upon the table exactly as he finds it in his book [Walls 1964].

Clarity characterized John Bell's publications, not least of all because of his accomplishments as an artist. In an artful metaphor, E.W. Walls (1964) writes that he renders polychromatic what had been monochromatic. Ruth Richardson (2009) finds Bell's realism extreme, and describes, "His dead are remnants of the human, meaty, mangled lumps cut to dangling shreds. Barely recognizable, human body parts lie awkwardly, in positions of unwarrantable intimacy and pain, hooks and chains claw and hold human skin, ropes suspend human joints, decapitated heads have faces with mouths agape, look agonized. Bell's dissecting room procedure without pity, or the slightest concession to human dignity." Though the illustrations are as stark as the rifling of bodies from the grave, which was their source material, Bell gave long-established facts a new significance and those that were nebulous a new clarity. He and his brother successfully used their artistic skills to get as much mileage as they could out of the sparse cadavers available in their day.

Henry Gray (1827–1861) and His Textbook

For a man whose name is a household word, this anatomist left few records of his life. Henry Gray was born, lived, and died a premature death in London. He studied at St. George's Hospital and was known

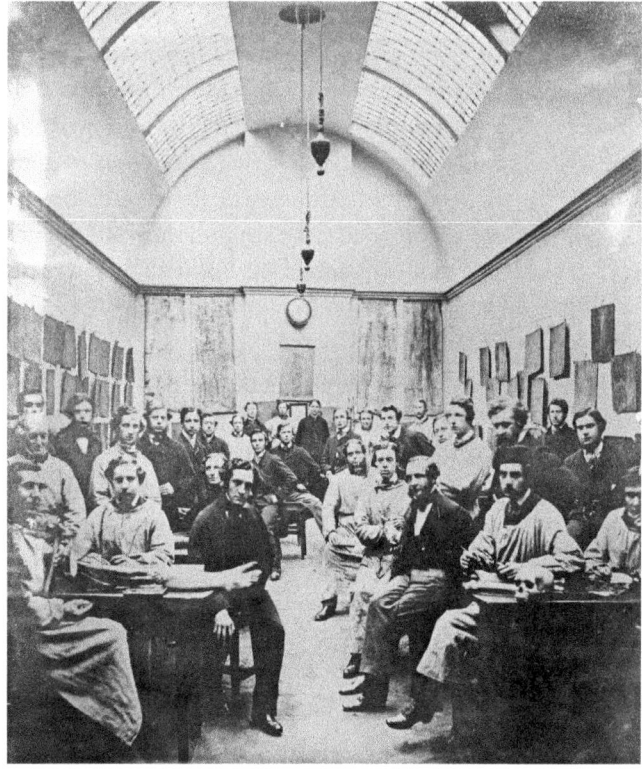

In this photograph of the dissecting room at St. George's Hospital, London, taken March 27, 1860, Henry Gray is seated next to the cadaver's feet. Anatomical prints are suspended on the walls and the room is lit from above by an arched skylight (*Wellcome Images*).

for being methodical and for learning anatomy by performing dissections himself, rather than merely observing anatomical demonstrations. His meticulousness paid off, and he was recognized for a paper on comparative anatomy of the eye by the Royal College of Surgeons while still a student. He won another prize, endowed by Sir Astley Cooper, for a 350-page dissertation on the spleen at the age of twenty-five, a year after he had been elected a Fellow of the Royal Society. Gray remained at St. George's after his studies as demonstrator of anatomy. He was then appointed curator of the museum, where his name remains attached to some of the specimens. Although the historic St. George's Anatomy Museum was destroyed during the Blitz, some original specimens survive. Gray preserved the heart of a twenty-five-year-old woman in solution because she had four rather than three aortic valve cusps, an anomaly that did not contribute to her death and had not even been detected during her life. The postmortem report of the woman with the heart defect exists in a bound volume, along with a case report of a man who fell fourteen feet, was paralyzed from the neck down, and died two days later. A portion of the unfortunate man's spine, showing the two separated cervical vertebrae that constituted his broken neck, remain where Gray placed it — on a bed of cotton in a glass vitrine.

Gray was promoted to St. George's lecturer of anatomy, a time-demanding post, and was later offered a position of assistant surgeon. Fittingly, one of the only two photographs of Gray to exist shows him seated at the foot of a corpse in a dissection room at St. George's Hospital crowded with teachers and students posed for the image. Always interested in anatomical research, Gray took the opportunity to observe the effects of smallpox at the bedside of his nephew Charles. Unfortunately, his curiosity proved deadly, despite his prior vaccination. He experienced an attack of the contagious disease, and it killed him. Gray was only thirty-four years old, but had left his mark.

Gray's legacy was his textbook, well-known for its clarity. Henry Gray collaborated with his younger colleague Henry Vandyke Carter, who was a gifted draughtsman and had provided illustrations for Gray's prize-winning dissertation. According to Gray's biographer (Hayes 2008), it was Carter who proposed the idea of an anatomy textbook, as he recorded in an 1850 diary entry, even though he had received no credit and only partial payment for the earlier project. Like Gray, Carter was a skilled anatomist, and together the two men put together a 750-page book with half as many labeled illustrations. Like Gray, Carter continued his teaching load while working on the book. The two probably did so on a daily basis, since dissection was a daytime and seasonal activity that was limited to the cooler weather of the school year. Carter could spend the summer months on sketching the skeleton and other specimens available in the museum.

Having been students and demonstrators themselves, Gray and Carter were well aware that the book needed to be clear and well-organized; it needed to be well-illustrated, yet affordable. Carter was able to bypass the process of having his drawings transferred in reverse onto wood blocks for printing by drawing mirror images of the anatomical structures directly onto the blocks themselves. The economy of their efforts is characterized by Gray's biographer:

> Between author and artist, there would be no wasted effort. Performing dissections together, for instance, would save time on many fronts, including helping them come to a speedy agreement on the fine points of each illustration—what stage of a dissection should be drawn, what perspective to use, and so on. As seasoned anatomists, too, they certainly knew how to make the most of their most precious resource, cadavers. Between dissections done for classes and those for the book, no material would go to waste [Hayes 2008].

In what may have been a shrewd political move, Gray dedicated the first edition of his book to St. George's most senior surgeon. He downplayed Carter's contribution, however, even though the useful and understandable illustrations—a fraction of which cited earlier anatomical works as inspirational—were in large part why this remarkably thorough contribution to the field was so very well-received. Upon the publication of Gray's *Anatomy Descriptive and Surgical* in 1858, the review in *The Lancet* was glowing:

> [W]e may say with truth, that there is not a treatise in any language, in which the relations of anatomy and surgery are so clearly and fully shown.... [I]t is impossible to speak in any terms excepting those of the highest commendation. The descriptions are admirably clear, and the illustrations, copied from recent dissections, are perfect [Hayes 2008].

Minor corrections were made and an index added to subsequent editions, but with these and perennial improvements the book is still in print more than 170 years later. The book has increased to more than double its original length under a series of envied editorships and has gone beyond morphology and systematic anatomy to serve today's students. Gray's *Anatomy* is now a classic, referred to in the advertising copy as "the granddaddy of all anatomy textbooks." The care put into the project by Gray and Carter ensured that it remains authoritative for medical students and informative for artists and interested laypersons.

Much of what made the anatomy text by Gray and Carter a success was their determination not to add artfulness to the presentation. Seated next to the cadaver, Carter declined to embellish or to include in his illustrations anything that was not relevant. Following Gray's written descriptions, which proceeded methodically through the body, Carter's drawings are vignettes of the relevant body parts. Kemp (2010) describes the style used throughout the book:

> The avoidance of any appealing views of the whole body — even the depiction of a complete skeleton — and his functional setting of the illustrations of the detailed parts of the body within the pages of printed text consistently negate any tendency to think that we are dealing with the "arty" production of a picture book. There is little modelling in light and shade, no attempt to place figures in graceful poses, and no evocative backgrounds. The whole book presents a heroically disciplined exercise in intellectual and visual restraint.... Its overt functionalism unequivocally exudes the air of institutionalized science instruction in the mid–19th century. As a consequence, it has a special style all of its own.

In no way could the book be seen as anything other than an educational tool to supplement the cadaver and assist anatomists and surgeons in learning their trade. Where other anatomists had translated the human body into a form that was both aesthetic and didactic — embalmer Frederik Ruysch in the seventeenth century and wax modeler Clemente Susini in the eighteenth, Henry Gray chose instead to transcribe rather than to translate. The to-the-point style of Gray's *Anatomy* was its artfulness.

3

Anatomists as Preparators and Collectors

It must have been a sight to see English surgeon William Cheselden out in the sunlight suspending part of a human skeleton from a tripod and then disappearing inside the curtained far end of a large rectangular box. Since it was likely the first time a camera obscura was used to capture medical images, the average eighteenth-century observer may not have known his purpose of translating the three-dimensional bones into two-dimensional drawings that could be reproduced in his textbook. The initiated, however, knew the beauty of his work and this included the medical students who assisted the anatomist and his illustrators. But these students and many others — not all of them with medical qualifications — saw not only the flat bones on the pages and the dry bones prepared for the sketches, but the raw, wet bones as they were first exposed in the cadavers Cheselden was able to procure. These observers may have been present at the anatomy theater where the well-respected doctor did some of his dissections or at his home where he was censured for doing others. Like Henry Gray, Cheselden and many other anatomists performed their dissections for a crowd *and* to prepare the still lifes and specimens that became the illustrations they presented to readers rather than a live audience.

For a certain subset of notable anatomists, dissections — whether public or private — were a means to an end. Their flourishes at the dissecting table, as deft as they may have been, were secondary to the specimens they produced from the bodies. Visitors were drawn from around the world to the anatomical cabinet of Frederik Ruysch in Amsterdam, the museum displays of Honoré Fragonard outside Paris, and the galleries of La Specola in Florence. The bodily preparations of Ruysch made such an impression on Russian czar Peter the Great that he purchased the entire set for the Kunstkamera he established his capital. The models made in the Italian workshop established by Felice Fontana so impressed Joseph II that the Austrian emperor commissioned his own set of anatomical waxes. The modelers had found that wax was the ideal medium for representing human flesh at about the same time the anatomists found that adding it to their well-guarded embalming formulae led to a lasting and aesthetically superior specimen. Pedagogical collections had been started in the seventeenth century when anatomists had begun to master preservation methods via arterial injection, which allowed them to retain the body parts they retrieved during dissections so that they could be used as teaching aids over and over again. But the cabinets of Ruysch and Fragonard went beyond the didactic.

Medical men were well aware that displayed anatomical collections needed to be well-preserved, practical, and — especially for the unprofessional audience — pleasing to the eye. Anatomists achieved lasting recognition through the proven preservation of their dissected specimens — tangible evidence of their talents, but a special few had a flair for presenting anatomical reality with a poetic or dramatic effect. Fragonard's preparations are called "lessons in medical anatomy, illustrations of artisanal virtuosity, and exercises in a distinctive macabre aesthetic" (Simon 2002). He positioned one flayed cadaver astride a skinless horse in an exercise that reads more as sculpture than a demonstration of comparative anatomy. Ruysch sculpted scenes in which to arrange his fetal skeletons, and positioned them in the midst of symbolic gestures. The resulting dioramas speak of the brevity of life rather than the physiological makeup of their tiny bones. The modelers of the anatomical waxes produced figures that conformed to standard images in the anatomical atlases of the day, but also created anatomical "venuses" that had hair, wore jewelry, and almost appeared to swoon. The waxes created in Italy stood out from those made in England because they appeared "alive" while the English models appeared "lifeless." The same distinction was made between Ruysch's vibrant wet specimens and the drab preparations on view at most medical museums. The result of such artifice in the preparation of anatomical specimens is an overlap of disciplines. "It has become a commonplace," writes Simon (2002), "to say that such anatomical preparations ... form a link between the worlds of art and science that are otherwise considered distinct."

In the disciplines of both art and science, nudity has been an accepted part of the presentation. Ruysch was not faulted for positioning a female infant in such a way that her gender could be neither mistaken nor overlooked. Simon (2002) points out the frank nudity in several of Fragonard's human figures, which contradicts the modesty demonstrated in the eighteenth century, when anatomical figures and illustrations were often cleverly contrived to hide the external sexual organs. In the eighteenth century and since, the educational value of such displays outweighed their prurience. As an example, a traveling exhibit of wax anatomical figures that toured France in 1712 had to adhere to sanctions imposed by Paris officials to uphold public decency. The collection had been organized by surgeon Guillaume Desnoies, who was ordered to limit the hours and some specific details of the display. Reading between the lines of the pronouncement, Simon (2002) speculates that Desnoies had included titillating sexual details — and perhaps real genitalia — on the models to draw the public into the exhibit. Even so, the show was allowed to continue its tour. Whether or not it was Fragonard's intention to use surprisingly sexual content to attract his audience, his embalmed cadavers and even the more demure wax venuses appealed to the voyeuristic.

Overt sexuality was not the only thing that lured visitors to anatomical displays in the eighteenth and nineteenth centuries, when "an explicit mission for public education served as a justification for combining anatomical figures with the perennial spectacle of prodigious diseases and monsters" (Simon 2002). For instance, the collection at the Athenaeum Illustre (now the University of Amsterdam) had been amassed over two careers in the nineteenth century and came to include more than two thousand human and animal specimens. It can be assumed that the majority of visitors over the years have come not to see the standard specimens prepared by Gerardus Vrolik, but to have a look at the human congenital anomalies preserved by his son Willem. Willem had been inspired by his father to teach anatomy, but focused his intense interest on teratology. He published books about cyclopia, conjoined twins, and other anomalies, and offered for display examples of human embryology, pathology, and puzzling and awe-inspiring "monsters." Also in Amsterdam, Ruysch knew the fascination that visitors had for monstrous births and, although he was just as proud of his teratology specimens, hid them behind his other specimens and brought them out upon request. Like the Vroliks, Ruysch and Fragonard preserved thousands of specimens, but chose to feature preparations that highlighted their skill rather than nature's oddities.

It was not deformities and it was much more than the genitals or the suggestion of sex that interested people in seeing these anatomical collections. To paraphrase Simon (2002), there is a tension between the ideal of detached scientific knowledge and the spectacular immediacy of the specimen as they appear before the viewer. The cabinets of anatomists who successfully exhibited their virtuosity in preserving or modeling anatomical specimens, provided educational tools that could be used to instruct medical students, *and did so in a dramatically compelling way* were added to the itinerary of international travelers and became a source of national pride. Ruysch displayed his moralizing tableaux of tiny animated skeletons atop his cabinets of more typical specimens, which drew attention to them. Fragonard kept his statuesque full-body preparations separate from the general specimens of comparative anatomy, and the deliberately dramatic presentation of his horse and rider was evidently intended to impress its audience just as much the piece's successful embalming (Simon 2002). Fragonard's contemporary, a royal veterinarian named Rumpelt who visited the collection in 1779, faulted him for just that, remarking that "the collection at Alfort was too much geared toward providing an attractive spectacle for a public that remained ignorant of innovations in anatomy-and thus that it had gained renown at the expense of scientific interest" (Simon 2002). The wide appeal of spectacular specimens is evidenced by the business these anatomists did in supplying private clients with specimens for their own cabinets.

These authentic and artistic specimens were incorporated into the natural history collections of the anatomists, their institutions, and their private clients, constituting an indispensable resource for the amateur and medical student alike. The flamboyance of certain specimens may not have added to their educational value, but has secured their historical value. As a whole, the permanent preservations — whether preserved bodies or wax facsimiles — stretched the limited resources of actual cadavers to dissect during student demonstrations. Preserved parts could be referred to in lecture, and the exhibits in medical museums could be consulted when classes were not in session. Observing the anatomical dissection, carried out before an audience by an experienced surgeon, was itself a vicarious introduction to human anatomy. A bit further removed were the written descriptions of the systems in the human body and the illustrations of the body's interior, drawn from life but necessarily presented in two dimensions. Between attending a dissection and consulting an anatomy textbook were alternatives, in wax and in the flesh.

Frederik Ruysch (1638–1731) and His Assemblages

Frederik Ruysch was an artful and accomplished Dutch anatomist who received his medical degree from the University of Leiden in 1661, was named professor of anatomy in 1662 (a position he held until his death), and in 1667 became praelector of the Amsterdam surgeon's guild. Ruysch made many anatomical discoveries during his career, taught botany, and was a forensic advisor to the Amsterdam courts. But it was his appointment in 1672 as chief instructor to the city's midwives that was most crucial to the anatomical legacy that he left. Through them, he had access to the bodies of infants which he preserved expertly and displayed in tableaux that were as highly thought of in his own day as they are today. Ruysch was both meticulous and prodigious when it came to preserving specimens for his cabinet. His work ethic is evidenced in a letter he wrote to his close friend in 1722: "Never does the sun rise too early for me, and nightfall always comes sooner than I could wish" (Mirilas et al. 2006). His hard work and great love for anatomy and dissection of the human body led to recognition throughout the world in the form of titles and awards from England, Prussia, France, and Russia. It also gained him plenty of private students willing to pay for the privilege of studying under the preparator of such a famed collection, even though Ruysch was never formally attached to a university as a professor of anatomy.

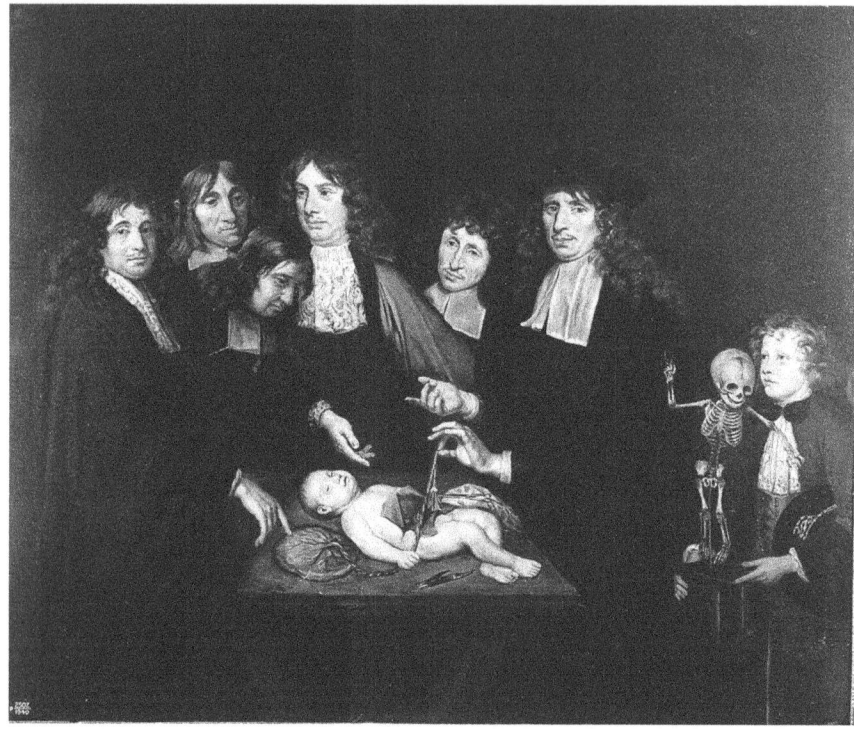

An early 20th century oil painting by B. F. Landis after a portrait by Jan van Neck, 1683, shows Frederick Ruysch (second from right), as praelector of anatomy, conducting a demonstration before the Amsterdam Guild of Surgeons. He lifts the umbilical cord of a dead child to show its connection between the infant's body and the placenta. The anatomist's son (far right) holds one of Ruysch's mounted fetal skeletons (*Wellcome Images*).

Ruysch was one of the first anatomists to preserve specimens by means of arterial embalming. He prepared thousands of wet specimens decanted in jars by injecting them with "liquor balsamicus," the ingredients of which he kept secret. The effectiveness of this fluid, which left the bodies looking astonishingly lifelike, is credited with transforming the messy business of dissection into a widely admired art. Ruysch's contemporary Bernard Le Bovier de Fontenelle wrote:

> All the bodies which he injected preserved the tone, the lustre, and the freshness of youth. One would have taken them for living persons in profound repose — their limbs in the natural paralysis of sleep. It

might also be said that Ruysch had discovered the secret of resuscitating the dead. His mummies were a revelation of life, compared with which those of the Egyptians presented but the vision of death. Man seemed to continue to live in the one, and to continue to die in the other [Hansen 1996].

Ruysch's carefully guarded professional secret involved the arterial injection of several fluids in succession. His medium to solidify the tissues probably included talc, white wax (or tallow), and cinnabar (red mercuric sulphide). His fluid to clear the vessels likely contained oil of lavender or turpentine. And the preservative fluid with which the specimens were injected, and in which they were immersed, may have been a large percentage of ethanol to which black pepper had been added (Roberts and Tomlinson 1989). Other additives, including colored pigments such as Berlin blue (also known as Prussian blue), were also used. His technique allowed him to overcome the color-loss issues, thereby imparting a living quality to dead flesh that left the wet specimens in medical museums looking pallid and lifeless. The bodies and organs that he prepared maintained their color and their shape.

A pink pigment would give the specimen a rosy flush of life which would not only cause it to retain a lifelike appearance after years or decades, but in a sense to allow it to live again. The anatomist boasted in the descriptions of specimens in his multi-volume *Thesaurus Anatomicus* that they remained fresh even twenty or thirty years since their deaths. This quality was also recognized by his contemporaries. An engraving that appears in one volume of the catalog depicts a skeleton recoiling in the presence of Ruysch's illuminated jars. A Latin verse attributed to Denis Papin reads in part: "Through thy art, O Ruysch, a dead infant lives and teaches and, though speechless, still speaks. Even death itself is afraid" (Hansen 1996). Ruysch excelled so well at reviving the dead that his skills were shown to frighten even the personification of death. De Fontenelle and many others considered Ruysch's preparations legitimate works of art. In bills of sale they were referred to as "precious and magnificent" artifacts and "artistic still lifes," and in catalogs of his work, Ruysch was consistently referred to as an artist rather than an embalmer (Hansen 1996). As Roberts and Tomlinson (1989) point out, "There is little need to emphasize the persistence of the somewhat obvious theme of 'inevitable fate' in anatomical illustration, but seldom has it been expressed in such a whole-hearted, enthusiastic, and extravagant way." With his exquisite delicacy, his anatomical assemblages far surpassed mere craftsmanship, as Hansen (1996) describes: "His skill in making tiny blood vessels, veins, and tissues approximate the flush of life was as magical as the skill required for the finest needlework."

Ruysch followed aesthetic principles with the intent of creating permanent examples he could draw from during his lectures — teaching aids that could be used again and again. The result was "a new aesthetic of anatomy that melded the acts of demonstration and display with the stylistic and emblematic meanings of vanitas art" (Hansen 1996). Prevented by civic regulations, Ruysch would never have been permitted to accumulate large numbers of adult bodies, and so was forced by circumstance to use the bodies of tiny fetuses and infants as the raw materials for his anatomical art. As "doctor to the court," he had access to the babies found drowned in the harbor, and others he obtained through his relationship to the city's midwives. But the multitude of baby bodies that he had at his disposal served his artistic purposes well. These little beings were innocent and untouched, but the tragedy of their unfulfilled lives gave them added poignancy as objects of contemplation, transforming their injected and decorated bodies into a new kind of still life (Hansen 1996). Of the more than six hundred specimens listed in Ruysch's catalog, at least a third are constructed from infants' bodies. A number of these were prepared in complete form, and the rest consist of partial preparations (mainly heads, arms, and legs). While ornamentation has been added to the remains of these children, they have been stripped of individual character. Instead of seeing them as specific subjects, these unfortunate infants and miscarried fetuses have been transformed into aestheticized objects of reflection, human materials that are to be viewed and valued only within the context of Ruysch's artistry (Hansen 1996).

Ruysch's specimens of infants, in whole or in part, allowing him to demonstrate his fine practical skills on the tiny bodies, in addition to his artistic sensibilities. They were paired with what, to the twenty-first century eye, seem like incongruous objects. The body of a female child, for instance, is placed on a fine brocaded pillow and holds a large tree of injected blood vessels, around which a delicate silk bow has been tied.

3. Anatomists as Preparators and Collectors (Frederik Ruysch)

Ruysch was assisted in his choices by his daughter Rachel, a still life painter, who helped him decorate the collection with flowers and shells, and dress the delicate body parts in lace and ornamental ribbons. Outfitting the babies with glass eyes gave them an animated gaze and a reanimated appearance (Hansen 1996). But dressing them was just as important:

> Moreover, the strategic placement of the clothing served a more important function than embellishment — it hid all discernible traces of dismemberment and embalming. Under the little sleeves and bonnets are the wide gashes of needles and the thick stitches of the embalmer's cord. By hiding the evidence of the reality of their death under layers of delicate infant wear, and by situating them within the sanctuary of the private cabinet of rarities, Ruysch was able magically to transform the anatomical body into an object of art [Hansen 1996].

But Ruysch went even further than this, setting up his infants in landscapes constructed not of bows and lace, but of cleverly utilized anatomical structures...

Kidney stones substitute for rocks, embalmed and hardened veins and arteries read as trees, intestines play the part of serpents and worms, and the tissue of lungs and other organs poses as shrubbery. Fetal skeletons stand among the organic components, holding handkerchiefs that are in fact preserved abdominal mesentery. Such are the tableaux of Frederik Ruysch, which no longer exist except in the detailed engravings by illustrator Cornelius Huyberts and written descriptions:

> Resting on a wooden base, the assemblage contains a number of piled-up gallstones and vascular trees, in one of the branches of which sits a stuffed bird; at the top stands a four-month-old human fetal skeleton. On either side of the assemblage are two other skeletons of similar age: one holds a tiny sickle; the other, in a pose of mourning, holds a handkerchief made of lung tissue up to one eye socket. "Why should I long for the things of this world?" reads the accompanying text, "Death spares no man, not even the defenseless infant" [Hansen 1996].

These dioramas, of which Ruysch created about twelve, were festooned with quotations emphasizing the brevity of life and the vanity of earthly riches. Through his preparations ran the theme of his day, *vanitas mundi,* the vanity of life coupled with the proximity of death. To this end, his tableaux were accompanied by inscriptions of Latin proverbs: "Vita humana lusus" ("Man's life is but a game"), "Vita quid est? Fumus fugiens et bulla caduca" ("What is life? A transient smoke and a fragile bubble"), and "Volat irrevocabile tempus" ("Time flies and cannot be recalled") (Mirilas et al. 2006). "By imbuing his specimens with vanitas symbolism," writes Hanson (1996), "Ruysch created tableaux vivants that thrilled his audience with their moving content. They also revealed scientific truths in an environment that countered his viewers' possible anxieties about death and dismemberment." The fetal skeleton described above bemoaning the value of worldly goods, grasps a string of pearls. Its companion plays a violin — an osteo-myelitic sequester with a dried artery for a bow, turns its eye sockets upwards, and whines, "Ah fate, ah bitter fate." More subtly, the tiny skeletal hands hold mayflies, which live only a single day in their adult state. The tableaux, with their memento mori symbolism, were depicted as being exhibited in Ruysch's museum atop the heavy wood and glass cabinets that contained his more standard — but still exquisite — medical specimens.

The purpose of Ruysch's artful preparations — scenes in which fetal skeletons played symbolic roles and infant limbs were dressed with dainty details — was to remove the sense of disgust that viewers experienced when looking at anatomical objects. He did this also by adding perfectly preserved appendages of children to jars containing the bone or organ of an adult, sometimes with a moralizing element. A small arm simply points to part of a lung dissected to show the thoracic nerves, but a baby's leg appears to kick the syphilitic skull of a prostitute. "The reason why part of the skull is placed under the little foot need not be sought far afield, since this prostitute would have not contracted this frightful disease had she not had such a reprehensible profession!" he wrote (Mirilas et al. 2006). Yet these were only a subset of his entire cabinet, as explained on the Kunstkamera (n.d.) website:

> Even today, anyone viewing his specimens realizes that this method works very well; it enables one to look into an open skull without nausea or without being repulsed. However, we have to realize that most of his other specimens, by far, were not ornamented with such special decorations and additions. The beautifully lace-decorated arms and legs had an important function for Ruysch and that is drawing the visitor's attention to other, smaller, anatomical specimens.

3. Anatomists as Preparators and Collectors (Frederik Ruysch)

But even with these, Ruysch went beyond the traditional by juxtaposing his specimens with natural materials. Thorns were used to direct the visitor's eye to a salient detail. A twig was placed to press a specimen against the glass of its container to make it easier to see. By achieving an unprecedented lifelike preservation and by using it and other non-objectionable items to direct the viewer's attention, Ruysch intended to enable his visitors to optimally immerse themselves in the anatomical knowledge he presented (Kunstkamera n.d.). As artful as it was employ gallstones as boulders in his little scenes, each had a clinical history that was recorded in his surgical notes.

One thing the anatomist *didn't* present, at least not as readily, was the anomalous, the aberrant, in the parlance of Ruysch's time, the monster. Many people — and their doctors — had believed since the sixteenth century that birth defects were caused when the sight of something frightening or horrific imprinted itself on the child in the womb of a pregnant woman. Ruysch questioned such interpretations, commenting on a specimen with a cleft lip, "On observing that such young creatures have allready such discomfort, one needs to consider if [it is correct] that in larger children their limbs, that were fine at first, were mutilated inside the body of their mother, from fright or from witnessing some spectacle?" (Driessen and Radzyun n.d.). He left it to others to reason why and how, restricting himself to describing and preserving the occasional misshapen infant. Ruysch displayed his teratology on less visible shelves in his cabinet or otherwise somewhat obscured. He did not want to frighten or upset the public. A child born with a single leg and several missing digits, for instance, was placed behind a bottle containing a normal child's small intestine. Other preserved deformities, such as a tiny fetus with a split palate and a harelip, were shown only upon special request. Though he took pains not to offend his patrons, the anatomist was as proud of his malformed specimens as he was of his normal preparations. Describing their vivid color in his catalogs, he deemed them a special pleasure for the eye (though he did question their true cause). Ruysch's expert embalming and his use of accessories made his monstrosities altogether different to the gaze than those exhibited in other medical museums, for which he judged other anatomists harshly. "It is better to bury such specimens than to exhibit them," he wrote (Kunstkamera n.d.).

It was his ability to preserve with such prowess, a passion inspired at the University of Leiden, where he studied side-by-side with another early arterial embalmer Jan Swammerdam, that allowed Ruysch to perform studies that required great precision and to make discoveries about minute structures including the tiny vessels of the lymphatic system, the skin, the brain, and the eye. The specimens in the anatomist's collection were definitively not just museum objects. They facilitated scientific study by himself and others, and served as materials to educate students. They were used as the basis of an eighteenth-century manual on ligaments that remains relevant even today (Driessen and Radzyun n.d.). So Ruysch's cabinet performed three-fold, functioning as a set of research specimens, a teaching collection, and an array of unique artworks.

> In the bodies that he prepared for public dissection and in the assemblages arranged for his cabinet at home, Ruysch created a wondrous stage, a theatrical and educational setting where his ideas could be demonstrated again and again.... To a modern eye, Ruysch's still lifes and preparations may appear nightmarish and bizarre. But to the seventeenth-century Amsterdam burghers, nobility, and medical professionals who visited his cabinet, such assemblages were wonderful, profound realities, and highly entertaining spectacles too [Hansen 1996].

Ruysch was as comfortable and adept on the floor of the anatomy theater as he was in the "theater" of his cabinet. Each of these stages represented a chance to share his knowledge by executing his skill and his artistry.

The post as Amsterdam's praelector of anatomy gave Ruysch income, prestige, and a setting in which to publicly dissect the anatomy he knew so well. He was the sole demonstrator at these ticketed performances, which — in addition to reinforcing his professional status within the circle of his peers — assumed the role of civic ritual. With only dim light admitted by the window, the anatomical theater was punctuated by lit scented candles, and was sometimes enhanced with flute music. The main event was the dissection of a human cadaver, but the price of admission paid for the banquet that would often follow, with a spread that included assorted dishes of meats, fish, and cakes, plus plenty of wine and tobacco. The anatomy lesson and its associated festivities drew laypersons to what was normally a restricted enterprise, but it was also attended by royalty and diplomats, and by scientists from abroad to whom it was publicized with the following invitation:

> Doctors of Medicine and Associates of the Faculty of Medicine, greetings to all who read this. By the favor of our distinguished magistrates I shall reveal to the sight of any of you who are curious to see what Nature has enshrined in all of us. Not out of a desire to vent malice on the work of God (the cadaver being that of an evildoer) but so that you may come to know yourself [Hansen 1996].

Ruysch relished his role as demonstrator, becoming the most active municipal anatomist in Amsterdam's history, having conducted some thirty-one public sessions during his lifetime.

Ruysch dissected the corpses of newly executed criminals and unclaimed bodies during his public demonstrations at the anatomical theater and private lessons he gave at his home. He performed more than one dissection of a pregnant woman, which allowed him to lecture on the anatomy of obstetrics. Ruysch's embalming allowed "bloodless dissection" (Hansen 1996), which eliminated many of the unpleasant aspects of anatomical study. The technique reduced the overpowering smell of decomposition, in addition to making the cadaver more aesthetically presentable. The anatomist was spared having to rush his demonstration, since the corpse could be prepared prior to the lesson and dissected over a matter of days. Dissection was no longer restricted to the colder months, and in fact Ruysch was the first anatomist in Amsterdam to perform public dissections during the summer (Hansen 1996). Even when fresh corpses weren't available, Ruysch was able to use cadavers he had previously preserved as examples of what he was discussing.

The anatomist's ability to prepare corpses for long durations is mentioned in a Dutch newspaper advertisement for a lesson he gave in 1695: "Mr. Frederick Ruysch will dissect on July 18 the body of a young boy who has been dead for well over two years" (Hansen 1996). For him, a fresh or embalmed body was preferable to teaching from books. Since 1696, Ruysch had been encouraging his colleagues to trust their own eyes in favor of the outdated manuals of ancient scholars. He offered his own specimens as proof of the discoveries he had made. He described and sketched them, but if that failed to convince, he invited doubters to his home. Ruysch had established his own private museum and extended his welcome: "Come and look ... let all come to me, on a clear day, no one will be refused to take a look" (Driessen and Radzyun n.d.). His anatomical cabinet, which filled five rooms, was open two days a week. By 1690, it was a popular tourist attraction. Among those who patronized it were philosophers, medical men, aristocrats, and royals. De Fontenelle described the wonder he experienced at viewing Ruysch one-of-a-kind collection: "His museum, or repository of curiosities, contain'd such rich and magnificent variety, that one would have rather taken it for the collection of a King than the property of a private man.... This museum was the admiration of foreigners: generals of armies, ambassadors, electors, and even princes and kings, were fond to visit it" (Hansen 1996).

One of these notables was Russian Czar Peter the Great, who toured the museum in 1697. Captivated by the beauty and allegory of the exhibits, Peter was drawn to the perfectly preserved body of a small child, who seemed to smile. Amazed, the czar is said to have leaned toward it and kissed the dead child's cold forehead. Czar Peter found that he shared many common interests with the Dutch anatomist beyond just surgery and anatomy. During the four months they spent together, Ruysch taught him how to collect and preserve butterflies, and how to pull teeth. Peter spent hours with the renowned Dr. Ruysch and found it hard to pull himself away from the cabinet and laboratory. He dined with Ruysch, and consulted with him about which surgeons had been chosen to return with him to attend the Russian troops. The czar admired Ruysch's knowledge and anatomical skill, and considered himself well-schooled under Ruysch's brief tutelage. On his second visit to Amsterdam, the czar greeted the anatomist warmly: "You are still my same old teacher" (Mirilas et al. 2006). It was on this visit in 1717 that Peter convinced Ruysch to part with his collection of curiosities for 30,000 guilders, an astronomical fee at the time. By importing Ruysch's collection, the czar had developed the interest in anatomy, which did not hold the philosophical, moral, theological, or aesthetic importance it held in Western Europe. The clinical approach of Russians toward anatomy continued (Driessen and Radzyun n.d.), but Frederik Ruysch was held up as a paradigm for all scientists of that era.

While Ruysch agreed to the sale of his famous cabinet, he refused to help with the packing and labeling, a task which took a month, and he immediately began amassing a new repository, which was sold after his death to the King of Poland, August the Strong. The specimens, divided between two ships, sailed the following year and arrived in Russia intact. They were installed at the Kunstkammer, the Russian Academy of Sciences' first public museum and anatomical theater. The Ruysch collection took its place in the cabinets along the perimeter of the round, bench-lined theater on the first floor. Word soon spread that St. Petersburg rivaled the European cities for the education of doctors and anatomists. A student there, H.F. Gross, wrote to a friend in Germany: "I am sure that if more German medical students would know about the possibilities for practical anatomical research here, they would prefer to come here, and for less money by way of Lübeck, than to go to Ruysch in Amsterdam, or to Paris" (Driessen and Radzyun n.d.). The anatomists of the Kunstkamera did research, prepared specimens, and gave lectures and anatomical lessons using cadavers at the meetings of the members of the Academy. While the historical record does not reflect who attended these public dissections, it is assumed that the crowd was made up mainly of scientists and students.

The 916 objects at St. Petersburg's Kunstkammer had finally begun to fade after nearly three centuries. A restoration project by the museum, with the participation of Dutch experts, was initiated in 2001. More than 200 of the wet specimens, which represent eighty percent of the collection, were treated and placed in new displays. Many of these had originally been placed in jars with narrow necks that had to be broken to extract and conserve the specimens. The dry specimens needed to be cleaned, and some of them required remounting of small fragments. While the restoration was being undertaken, experts began linking the preparations — dried specimens, embalmed organs and body parts, whole fetuses and neonates, and complete skeletons — with the original descriptions written by Ruysch himself and published in his *Thesauri*.

Survived by his specimens, Frederik Ruysch is also immortalized on canvas in the dissecting theater he filled so many times. Two portraits of the anatomist/artist exist, both entitled "Anatomy Lesson of Dr. Frederik Ruysch." The works hung with five others — including Rembrandt's "Anatomy Lesson of Dr. Nicolaas Tulp"— in the formal meeting rooms of the Amsterdam surgeons' guild headquarters. This was where the public anatomical demonstrations were held, and where junior barber-surgeons and midwives were examined and certified. One canvas was painted by Adriaen Backer in 1670 and depicts Ruysch demonstrating the inguinal canal on the left thigh of an adult cadaver. The dissection was conducted over a period of five days in the month of March, and like all official dissections was attended by guild members, magistrates, city governors, and members of the interested public. A youthful Ruysch flays the leg delicately, surrounded by six of his colleagues. The artistic license employed in documenting historical events like this allowed for the alteration of the sequence, in which the extremities would have been the last parts of the body to be exposed. The names of three of these surgeons, who paid to be included in the painting, can still be read as inscriptions on the right pilaster. The presence of the statues of the Greek gods of medicine, Apollo and Asclepius, paid homage to them while creating a striking visual contrast between the ancients and their modern counterparts, the medical men of the seventeenth-century (Hanson 1996). The grandeur and theatricality of the scene elevated the status of both anatomy and the guild representing its practitioners.

This holds true of the other canvas, painted by Jan van Neck in 1683, which shows a more mature Ruysch anatomizing the blood vessels of the umbilical cord and placenta of a preserved infant. On the far right of the painting stands a young boy holding an infant's prepared skeleton, possibly intended as an artistic device to bridge the age gap between the babies and the adults (Hansen 1996). The boy is identified in guild records as the anatomist's son Hendrik, who was actually several years older at the time. The black brimmed hat he holds — identical to that of his father — may signify his anatomical lineage. Because there is no dissection of an infant's body in the official records for 1683, it is assumed that this painting was not sponsored by the guild, but commissioned by Ruysch himself. Hanson (1996) reasons that the later painting improves on the earlier portrait: the canvas is larger, standing up better against Rembrandt's painting of Dr. Deyman, whom Ruysch had succeeded; the anatomist appears more confident and is more prominent in the composition; and the subject being dissected is an infant, which plays to Ruysch's strengths.

Both painters Backer and van Neck, like Rembrandt, used a dark palette and dramatic lighting to heighten the drama and intimacy of the scene. But unlike the cadaver in "The Anatomy Lesson of Dr. Nicolaes Tulp," which exhibits rigor mortis, blackened lips and toes, and sallow skin, the bodies being dissected by Ruysch appear fresher and without signs of putrefaction. "With their flushed skin tones and languid poses, the corpses depicted in the two pictures appear more like sleeping or swooning patients on surgery tables than dead bodies subjected to dissection," writes Hanson (1996). There is no evidence of the violence (hanging) that ended the life of the criminal Joris van Iperen, who lies on the dissecting table painted by Backer. In addition, the size of the infant in van Neck's painting is exaggerated to point to its importance in the image as it relates to Ruysch's role as dissector and preparer (Hansen 1996). Both paintings can be read as nods to the mastery of the anatomist's mastery of embalming techniques — a mastery that can still be observed in the hundreds of specimens that remain to exemplify it.

William Cheselden (1688–1752) and the Skeleton

William Cheselden was born in Somerby, Leicestershire, England, and given a classical premedical education. At the age of fifteen, he was apprenticed to a local surgeon, but soon moved to London, where he studied under anatomist William Cowper and St. Thomas's Hospital surgeon James Ferne. At the age of twenty-two, Cheselden began lecturing on anatomy at St. Thomas's. His syllabus listed thirty-five lectures repeated four times per year. He had been admitted to the Company of Barber-Surgeons, but the popularity of his lectures interfered with the routine instruction given at Barber-Surgeons Hall. The need for concentrated anatomical coursework within the medical profession prompted him to offer classes in his home, dissecting privately the few bodies of executed prisoners that the company was allotted. This brought him into conflict with the barber-surgeons, whose mild censure is recorded in their minutes:

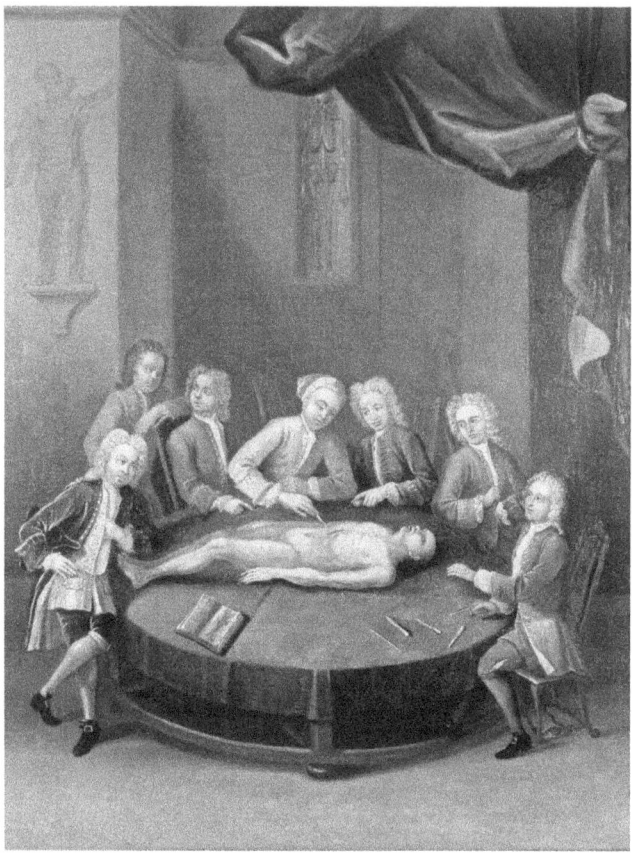

This scene painted circa 1730 or 1740 shows renowned English surgeon William Cheselden performing a private dissection in the anatomy theater of the Barber-Surgeons' Company in London for the benefit of six spectators. The men are either Cheselden's colleagues or a group of interested gentlemen (*Wellcome Images*).

At a Court of Assistants of the Company of Barbers and Surgeons held on March 25th, 1714; our Master acquainting the court that Mr. William Cheselden, a member of this Company, did frequently procure the dead bodies of malefactors from the place of execution and dissect the same at his own house, as well during the Company's public lectures as at other times without the leave of the Governors and contrary to the Company's by-law in that behalf; by which means it became more difficult for the beadles to bring away the Company's

3. Anatomists as Preparators and Collectors (William Cheselden)

> bodies, and likewise drew away the members of this Company and others from the public dissections and lectures at the Hall. The said Mr. Cheselden was thereupon called in, but having submitted himself to the pleasure of the Court with a promise never to dissect at the same time as the Company had their lecture at the Hall, nor without leave of the Governors for the time being, the said Mr. Cheselden was excused for what had passed, with a reproof for the same pronounced by the Master at the desire of the Court [Archæologica Medica 1898].

Cheselden was well-respected and was allowed to continue his anatomy demonstrations at St. Thomas's and at his home. He became surgeon at St. George's Hospital when that institution was founded in 1733. Years later, shortly after he had been elected Warden of the Company of Barber-Surgeons, Cheselden led other London surgeons to break with their barber fellows in a successful bid for professional recognition. In 1745, they formed their own Company of Surgeons, which later evolved into the Royal College of Surgeons of England.

Remembered by urologists for the rapid removal of bladder stones through a surgical procedure he developed, Cheselden is associated by anatomists with the skeleton, which he documented in *Osteographia*, the first life-sized and accurate description of every bone in the human body. An unprecedented atlas of osseous anatomy, the book captured the details of crocodile, bear, ostrich, and other animals in a section on comparative anatomy; descriptions of diseases of the bone; and the structure of the human skeletal system. Cheselden achieved this by using — and possibly designing his version of — a camera obscura. Precursor of the photographic camera. this was a darkened box equipped with a lens at one end and the artist positioned at the other end to trace the image projected by a designated object placed outside the box in direct sunlight. Cheselden's student published a description of the apparatus and its use:

> It is a long square Tube set upon two Tressels ... whose Inside is made black, to prevent the Reflection of Light; towards that End which is nearest the Object, is a Convex Glass placed in a sliding Frame, thro' which the Rays passing from the Object, converge and meet in a Focus upon the Table-Glass placed near the other End, analagous [sic] to the Crystalline Humour and Retina in the Eye. The Object here represented is the Trunk of a Skeleton fix'd to a Painter's Ezel, which being inverted, appears upright on the Table-Glass, on the rough Side of

which the Artist delineates with a Pencil, which afterwards he traces off on Paper. The Convex Glass placed in the sliding Frame being moved backward or forward, makes the Object bigger or less, keeping its due Proportions. This Camera has several Advantages beyond the common one; for in this, Objects as big as the Life may be taken, or reduced gradually to any Scale; whereas the other only diminishes, and that in a very great Degree [Neher 2010].

Probably the first person to use a camera obscura for medical imagery, Cheselden includes an image of it on the title page of *Osteographia*, thereby asserting to his readers that the illustrations were objective translations of three-dimensional skeletons into two dimensions. The artistic grace was achieved in the composition and perspective.

Though he was said to have been a competent draughtsman, Cheselden employed two artists, Gerard van der Gucht and Jacob Schijnvoet, to make the initial drawings. In his prefatory remarks addressed to the reader, he takes full responsibility for the process which he oversaw and the results which he approved: "The actions of all the sceletons [sic] both human and comparative, as well as the attitudes of every bone, were my own choice: and where particular parts needed to be more distinctly expressed on account of the anatomy, there I always directed; sometimes in the drawings with the pencil, and often with the needle upon the copper plate, and where the anatomist does not take this care, he will scarce have his work well performed" (Neher 2010). With his artists and his students under his direction — and with what must have been an ample and envied collection of animal and human bones — Cheselden arranged the suspension (necessarily upside-down) of each skeletal subject from the three-legged easel set up at the perfect distance from the lens. One can then imagine him at the shoulder of the artist seated in the far end of the shrouded box as they adjusted the glass plate to begin the drawing. As Neher (2010) writes, "He needed their artistic skills to create images of the highest quality and they needed his anatomical knowledge to understand what they were making images of."

Cheselden's osteography- subtitled *The Anatomy of the Bones*— is assessed to be an even greater achievement than his first major work, *The Anatomy of the Humane Body*, which became a standard medical textbook for nearly one hundred years. Published in 1713, it remained in print through sixteen English and American editions. Among other departures from the anatomy texts of the day, Cheselden's *Anatomy* was written in English rather than the traditional Latin. With forty leaves of plates, it was admired for its artistic illustrations as well as its scientific merit, and no doubt required a prodigious number of anatomical dissections to achieve. It is his books which survive him. The only holdings associated with the great anatomist at the Royal College of Surgeons are not the skeletons that were reproduced on their pages, but papers detailing his agreements with his publishers. Cheselden is remembered in a painting from approximately 1730 in which he conducts a dissection in Barber-Surgeon's Hall for the benefit of a group of his colleagues or interested gentlemen.

Clemente Susini (1757–1814) and the Anatomical Waxes

Technically, Clemente Susini was not an anatomist. But he worked side-by-side with one for the forty years during which he was employed at the Museum of Physics and Natural History in Florence. Better known as La Specola, the museum was one of the centers of the eighteenth-century talent for anatomical wax modeling. Wax likenesses of anatomical dissections offered a more durable alternative to the relatively unsuccessful attempts to preserve the actual dissected specimens by means of injection. The necessity of anatomists in training to have to dissect and examine unpreserved dead bodies, coupled with the difficulty of obtaining them at all, meant overcoming revulsion or confining the demonstrations to the winter months. There were early attempts by Italian physician Marcello Malpighi and Dutch naturalist Jan Swammerdam to address the problem by arterially injecting preservative fluids composed of alcohol, different metals (including mercury, lead, tin, and bismuth), wax, and sometimes coloring agents. But in time, these embalmed bodies deteriorated. An alternative method of providing an accurate reproduction of the various organs of the human body was clearly required (Ballestriero 2010), and wax models served this need.

The dream of Felice Fontana, founder of the Florentine school of anatomical modeling, was indeed to create anatomical models of scientific value for teaching purposes while removing the sense of repulsion produced by cadavers (Ballestriero 2010). Wax models were not created with the sole intention of *representing* anatomical parts, but of *replacing* them (de Ceglia 2005). They allowed physicians to learn anatomy without getting their hands dirty. Fontana's studio aimed at reproducing the entire human anatomy down to the smallest detail visible to the unaided eye. Modeled on actual cadavers, the wax medium conveyed reality but was reassuringly artificial. Even so, Fontana intended them to comprise a comprehensive three-dimensional anatomical atlas. To this end, and to ensure that the collection of anatomical waxes they were building could serve their didactic purpose with or without a guide, he supplemented the models with colored drawings above the appropriate display case and included annotated watercolors and detailed instructions in the corresponding drawer underneath (Ballestriero 2010). But even without consulting the additional explanatory information, including the correct term for each anatomical detail (Schnalke 2004), students were supposed to be able to see with the utmost clarity how even the most fragile structures of the body functioned.

As important to the production of the anatomical waxes at La Specola was their finished presentation. Although attention was explicitly directed to a vast number of bodily fragments, the main intention behind the studio's attempts at three-dimensional representation was always to summarize: to provide an overview of the body's details as parts of a whole (Schnalke 2004). Fontana arranged the display cases in a series of spacious rooms, with functionally related areas of the body adjacent to one another. As visitors directed their attention to smaller and smaller structures, it was expected that when they looked back up at the room they would regain the sense of the body as an integral unit. The rhythm of the exhibit had been meticulously worked out, from the arrangement of numerous wax studies of body parts, to representations of larger functional body systems, and — most often in the center of the room — to life-size models of whole figures (Schnalke 2004). Today, the ten-room exhibit at La Specola still stands as the largest collection of anatomical waxes in Europe. And even now the eyes move as intended between individual organs, such as the series on the anatomy of the heart, and the many full-bodied specimens, such as "The Skinned Man," a recumbent male figure demonstrating the musculature.

Fontana set up the La Specola workshop probably towards the end of 1771 (Azzaroli 1977), hiring Giuseppe Ferrini to do the wax modeling. The dissections, at first carried out by Fontana himself, were soon taken over by anatomist Paolo Mascagni, whose lectures had made him very popular and marked Florence as an anatomical center despite its lack of a university. In 1773, a teenage Clemente Susini was brought in to the workshop as a modeler. Susini had been born and raised in Florence. He was schooled as a sculptor (later becoming a member of the city's Academy of Fine Arts). Five years after he had begun his apprenticeship, Susini — then twenty-five years old — was appointed chief modeler. But under the authoritarian direction of Fontana, who personally inspected all waxes produced in La Specola workshops, Susini and his fellow modelers were probably allowed very little artistic latitude despite the full potential of the medium. The wax could be tinted directly, permitting the achievement of the perfect imitation of nature. Because of its transparency, wax also reproduced the opalescence and delicacy of human flesh. This added a tactile quality further enhanced by lifelike poses (Lemire 1992). It was only after Fontana's death in 1805 that Susini and the others began claiming ownership of their creations, and brought the Florentine art of wax modeling to the highest peak of artistic perfection (Ballestriero 2010). Until then, they carried out Fontana's vision, which grounded them in human anatomy and in the nuances of their wax medium, with which they were ingenious at making the internal workings of the body understood.

The craft was not only labor-intensive for both modeler and anatomist, each model required the use of a number of dissected cadavers. It was said that some of the models required the study of up to two hundred corpses (Schnalke 2004). As the staff in Florence increased, they were organized into teams, with their duties strictly defined. The anatomist determined the design of the projected model, and supplied the artists in the wax studio with images and, more anatomist the exact part of the body to be shown, how the body or body part was to be posed, how the section fit into the whole, and other details. Highly specialized production tasks were carried out by certain modelers and their assistants, with production a carefully orchestrated process. The wax figures were created by plaster casting the organs of a cadaver directly to make the molds into which wax was poured in successive layers at different temperatures. Structures that could not be reproduced in this way were sculpted in the wax, which was a mixture of melted beeswax, animal fat, plant oil, and dye. Arteries, veins, and nerves were created with thread or wire dipped in wax. The models were reinforced by iron supports. For efficiency, prototypes developed were that could be varied as necessary to allow the workshop to output models on a massive scale.

In 1793, a medical officer to the Napoleonic armies in Italy, spent nearly a year at La Specola and left an invaluable written record of the wax modeling technique used by the Florentine School. Dr. De Genettes wrote:

> Most of the organs represented by colored waxes are cast in plaster moulds formed directly from the natural organs. The finishing touches are then added by a skilled sculptor who works side-by-side with the actual cadaver. The sculptor always works under the supervision of an anatomist, because even the most excellent sculptors would be unable to reproduce nature accurately without such guidance. Any organs that cannot be cast directly are modelled in clay or wax by artists who are extremely skilled in this type of work and copy from the cadaver itself. A plaster impression is then cast on these models. This technique is used particularly for statues of whole figures. When a plaster cast is to be made for an anatomical statue, a sculptor is firstly commissioned to produce a full size wax model. This is copied from life, nude and in the position the anatomist finds that the organs or parts to be represented are shown to the greatest effect. This first stage takes about six months. When complete, separate models of individual organs must be made once each has been dissected; and the entire process must be carried out under constant supervision and guidance.

To break it down, the production process was carried out in four stages, described below.

The first stage involved sectioning a human cadaver under the supervision of an expert dissector. This was done to isolate the organs and structures that were to be reproduced in wax. Before proceeding to the next stage, the wax used to model the anatomical parts was prepared. A mixture was made that incorporated wax from bees and other insects, including plant parasites. The blend was poured into a large tin-plated copper cauldron. As the wax mixture melted over a very low heat, lard and sperm oil (or plant oil) were added to the mixture until it reached the right consistency. During the second stage, molds were cast directly from the cadaver or a specific anatomical structure. After coating the body or body part with a protective layer of fat, the plaster was applied. This would form negative impressions that would be kept to reuse so that the same piece could be reproduced over and over again without having to be recast. The third stage involved producing the model in colored wax, which required both delicacy and artistic skill. Dye that had been dissolved in turpentine was added to the heated wax. Small quantities of natural dyes including cinnabar and granulated white wax were added when needed to obtain the required muscle or organ color. The plaster cast was soaked in warm water and its inner surface was spread with soft soap to make it less porous so that the model would release easily. The heated and colored wax mixture was then poured into the mold in successive layers, with each at layer applied at a progressively lower temperature. After the poured wax had sufficiently cooled, the mold was opened. The model could then be finished in the fourth and final stage. Any imperfections in the wax were scraped away, and the surface of the model was polished with a soft brush soaked in oil of turpentine. Muscle striations were carved into the wax using heated iron implements of various shapes and sizes. Structures such as membranes were either painted or imitated using thread. Arteries, veins, and nerves were produced using wax-coated wire or thread. The finer vessels were added with a very fine paintbrush and additional colors were painted in as required. Lastly, the surface of the model was coated in clear varnish, which muted the colors, added a luster that gave it the illusion of living tissue, and also protected it from dust.

    One early advancement of Susini's renown was his participation in filling the commission Fontana had received from Joseph II of Austria. The emperor had admired both the aesthetic qualities and medical usefulness of the wax models on a visit to the La Specola museum in 1780. Eager for Vienna to have such a collection, he arranged the following year to have a set made by Fontana's modelers. The work was carried out over the next five years under Mascagni's scientific supervision. The impressive total of some eight hundred models was transported across the Alps in wicker baskets loaded on the back of mules, then floated down the Danube by boat. The journey caused some of the models to break, and others to crack from the cold, but when the bulk of these anatomical waxes was exhibited in the Josephinum for the benefit of medical students in Vienna, they were met with great acclaim. They are still on display and are described on the website Curious Expeditions (2007):

> The models are magnificent. They are near-perfect three-dimensional representations of the human body. Many models are simply parts of the whole: the muscles of an arm, different parts of a lung, the bones of a shoulder, a heart handsomely mounted under a glass dome. But some are complete bodies, with parts exposed down to the bone, or to the muscle, or to just under the skin, many with waxen eyes wide open. Some are laying in glass display coffins on a bed of silk like Snow White. Some are posed, seemingly writhing in agony. Others are upright in tall standing cases. One model ... has long flowing hair and a dainty set of pearls, [and] can be completely disassembled by students.

So many of the waxes have survived that they are arranged — still in their original rosewood cases — in a series of three rooms.

In addition to entire collections created for La Specola between 1771 and 1893, numerous projects were undertaken at the famous Florence workshop. Models of both normal and diseased anatomical parts, and specialized series of human and plant specimens for obstetricians and botanists, were made for universities throughout Europe. Waxes were shipped to universities and museums within Italy (Turin, Pavia, Genoa, Pisa, Siena, and Perugia), in France and Switzerland, and as far afield as Egypt. Susini, in particular, was singled out for many of the commissions that followed the studio's patronage by Joseph II. He was paid by staff anatomist Paolo Mascagni to model his numerous discoveries about the lymphatic system. He was also hired by Francesco Antonio Boi, chair of Anatomy at the University of Cagliari in Sardinia, to create what became known as the "Cagliari waxes." Created between 1803 and 1805, the models in the collection represent a turning point in Susini's style. Where the Florentine waxes had come to resemble "lavish dolls" (Ballestriero 2010), the waxes sent to Sardinia were lifeless, with glazed eyes and pallid cheeks. But new to the Cagliari collection was the fact that each of the models was unique. The facial features were not made to resemble idealized human beings, but were real portraits. Each wax sculpture, for which a considerable sum was paid at the time, was signed and dated. The identification of the wax-workers at La Specola — unlike the many anonymous artists at other workshops — as the producers of certain models, elevated their status as artists. It meant that Susini's name has been remembered for the centuries that his wax creations have remained extant. At Cagliari, this necessitated a careful restoration by the University's chair of anatomy Luigi Cattaneo in the 1960s, since the waxes had been wrapped in newspaper and hidden during World War II, but these, like the models at La Specola, can still be seen today.

What Susini and the Florentine modelers remain best known for are their "Venus" figures. The partially-dissected anatomical waxes of reclining women came to be known by this reference to the "Venus de Medici," a Roman copy of an ancient Greek statue on display in Florence's Uffizi Gallery and well-known since the seventeenth century. The wax models imitated not only the body, but classical sculpture that had become representative of classical beauty. Susini's "Medici Venus" was so highly regarded — for both its aesthetic and educational value — that his contemporaries in anatomical museums all over Europe ordered copies. The figure produced for display in the La Specola collection was reproduced in different sizes and postures for numerous clients in Italy in other countries, including Spain, Austria, and Hungary (Ballestriero 2010). With her head thrown back and her arms open, the "Medici Venus" — and many of the other female wax models in La Specola — gives the appearance of a beautiful woman in her death throes. In describing the version of Susini's Venus at the Semmelweiss Museum of the History of Medicine, de Ceglia (2005) characterizes the fate of the female cadaver under the medical gaze: "In the Budapest version, the right leg is slightly raised, as if in a last attempt to conceal what will be examined shortly after with sadistic and voyeuristic glee." In fact, the scholar (de Ceglia 2005) notes slight variations in each of the copies Susini produced. The Bologna Venus hangs her head and seems to be on the brink of collapse.

The Venus in Vienna turns her eyes away as if she is afraid to look at her torturer.

All of the full-body female waxes produced in Florence seem to be aware of their fate, prompting de Ceglia (2005) to characterize them as "conscious sacrificial lambs on a dissecting-room table." Like the funerary sculptures on Renaissance tombs, their expressions hover between agony and ecstasy. Susini's Venus is sensual without being overtly sexual. Visitors were invited to admire the Medici Venus's external form, while then being allowed to dismantle her piece by piece. When the wax sculpture was viewed by French portraitist Madame Vigée Lebrun in 1792, she was shocked: "That sight made such an impression upon me that I nearly fainted. For several days I could think of nothing else, to such an extent that I failed to look at anyone without mentally stripping them of clothes and skin" (de Ceglia 2005). But what is even more stunning than her barely suppressed sexuality is her highly concealed pregnancy! Though she does not have an enlarged abdomen, heavy breasts, or any of the other typical indicators, her removable uterus hides a fetus. The outward signs of gestation are ignored in favor of portraying the ideal female form, one instance in Susini's workshop of art trumping science.

The pearl necklace that the Medici Venus is wearing is seen by some as accentuating her nudity, and by others as symbolic of her vanity. For scholar Thomas Schwalke, it is a sign of her individuality. Rather than *vanities*, he sees the gestures of the partially dissected Venuses and the other models in the La Specola collection as *vanitas*:

> Such distractions of the scientific gaze are most apparent when we look at elements related to the theme of vanitas or memento mori, which had already figured in anatomical illustrations of the seventeenth century and which were included in the foremost scientific textbooks until well into the enlightened eighteenth century. In the same vein, some of the Florentine wax figures seem to be still alive, or rather to be lamenting their death post festum, from beyond the grave. Some of the whole figure models, as well as numerous studies of functional details where the head is included as a motif, show not only body parts such as eyes, ears, nose, mouth and hands — i.e. features which determine the body's individual expression — they also often feature intact body surfaces not cut away by the scalpel. A number of models even have artificial eyes and human hair and are sometimes adorned with ornaments like a

pearl necklace, and some are placed on decorative lace and satin cushions [Schnalke 2004].

The wax medium gave the models the appearance of living skin, but the expert sculpting of Susini and the other Florentine modelers gave the figures the semblance of life. The areas where the skin has not been sectioned to reveal the underlying tissue, in combination with the external accessories, allow the viewer to experience the Medici Venus as if she were alive — and not just a medical patient, but a coy female.

Some believed that the scientific purposes for creating the anatomical waxes were just an excuse for depicting beautiful, sensual dying women. The male waxes, in contrast, were presented with no eroticism. They, too, had features reminiscent of classical statues, but their eyes are dispassionate, their sexual organs are openly but plainly displayed, and they are shown without skin, hair, or accessories (de Ceglia 2005). But it was the beauty of the female anatomical waxes that drew praise. Even relatively early on, during a visit to La Specola during his first Italian tour in 1786, German writer Johann Wolfgang von Goethe recognized the symbiosis of art and science that the Florentine waxes represented. He was enthusiastic about the collection, and although he was unsuccessful at lobbying for establishing a collection in Berlin, he was convinced that didactics and aesthetics went hand in hand (Schnalke 2004). Medical men clamored for Susini's models because they combined absolute precision with artfulness. He represented the latest discoveries in anatomy as realistically as possible, but he conveyed them with a sensuality informed by the beginnings of the Romantic movement. Such was the visual appeal of many of his models that they were not only used for educational purposes but were sought by private collectors and museums. His wax cadavers were beautiful. His science was art. This was recognized by both the scholars and sculptors of the time. Adolph Murray, anatomy professor at the University of Uppsala, praised the exactitude of his work. Famous Italian sculptor Antonio Canova commented favorably on his artistic abilities. When he died, Susini's obituary praised "the beauty which he gave to the most revolting things" (Museo dello Cere Anatomiche n.d.). The wax work at La Specola fell to students whom he had trained and mentored, but the consensus was that they didn't have the talent of their mentor.

Under Clemente Susini's guidance, however, the Florence school of wax anatomical modeling as a whole had surpassed the Bologna school from which the art had spread. In fact, a number of Florentine waxes — including an example of Susini's Venus — are curated in Bolognese museums, even though wax models had been concurrently produced in that city. Following Bologna's example of using wax to reproduce anatomical specimens, similar studios had been set up in some of the leading universities in other European cities, but few examples of these early eighteenth-century waxes have survived. One thing that set the Florentine models apart was their style. Frankfurt physician Engelbert Wichelhausen, who visited La Specola in 1794, states that the anatomists were instructed to dissect bodies to make them look like the well-known engravings in published works on anatomy. In this way, the wax models were made to conform to standard images available in anatomical atlases of the period (Panzanelli 2008). Of course, the anatomy illustrations of the time were very artful. This leaves a striking comparison between the aesthetic models crafted at La Specola and the more clinical models produced at the University of Bologna.

The first anatomical waxes were produced in Bologna in the 1690s, through collaboration between the Sicilian artist Gaetano Giulio Zumbo and French surgeon Guillaume Desnoues. Their joint endeavor resulted in the creation of the first realistic anatomical models made from colored wax, resulting in a valid alternative to dissected human specimens that was both realistic and long-lasting. Zumbo (also spelled Zummo) was an abbot, whose spirituality is believed to have been the motivator for his creation of waxworks of a predominantly religious nature. He later became fascinated by death and disease, which materialized in gruesomely realistic depictions. His highly realistic tableaux — "The Plague," "The Triumph of Time," "The Vanity of Human Glory," and "The Syphilis" — are known collectively as the "Theatres of Death," and convey the fragility of life and the decay of disease. These and an anatomical head modeled by Zumbo are on display at La Specola Museum. Unlike the graceful models produced at the Florence workshop, these earlier works are explicitly macabre, and portray destruction in minute detail and with a morbid attention to its trivial aspects (Ballestriero 2010).

The seventeenth-century head by Zumbo in the collection at La

Specola is the earliest surviving anatomical wax model explicitly created for medical didactic purposes. The head, which bleeds from the nose and mouth, was likely patterned after that of an executed man. The blood, which was considered by later anatomical wax modelers to be taboo, was intended to be symbolic of the human condition. The signs of decay horrify modern viewers, but impressed Zumbo's contemporaries with their fidelity. The features and exposed teeth give an appearance of a grimace and show, along with some of the other models, stylistic elements typical of contemporary late–Baroque sculpture. These same elements fit the eighteenth century's morbid, Gothic idea of artistic beauty. Their appeal was extolled by the Marquis de Sade, after he saw the waxes on a visit to Italy:

> In this hall, a bizarre idea came to life: a tomb full of corpses at different stages of putrefaction, from the moment of death till the complete destruction of the individual.... The impression created by this masterpiece is so strong that each sense seems to trigger alarm to the others. You bring your hand to your nose as an automatic reaction [de Ceglia 2005].

By the nineteenth century, opinions about what constituted artistic beauty — along with the public's attitude toward death — changed. The waxes by Zumbo, so eerily redolent of decay, were considered perverse and pornographic. They fell out of favor, but were held in the collections in Florence and Bologna.

Retained to this day at the University of Bologna's Museo Delle Cere Anatomiche "Luigi Cattaneo" are waxes representative of that school's clinical style. Nineteenth-century modelers Giuseppe Astorri and Cesare Bettini worked with anatomists Francesco Mondini, Luigi Calori, and Cesare Taruffi to produce anatomical wax models of normal morphology, but also to reproduce variations, malformations, abnormalities, and morphological alterations. Moulages, waxes showing injuries or pathological changes in the body, had begun to circulate in traveling shows across Europe. Serving partly as entertainment and partly as public health education, they often featured the effects of sexually transmitted diseases. Similar to Fontina adding to the educational value of his waxes by providing annotated illustrations, the anatomy professors at Bologna preserved, whenever possible, the anatomical specimen of the case under pathological examination so that it could be displayed next to the corresponding wax model. These sets, as well as drawings that were also preserved, provided medical students with valuable information and leave us with a full picture of the methods of the anatomists of the time. What we know of the modelers, at least those in Susini's time, is that they used natural skeletons as a base for their full-body models, consequently they took longer to produce and were more expensive than those made by the Florentines.

The wax models produced in England and the northern European countries had a very different look than those made in Italy — whether the fluidity of the Florentines or the more literal interpretations from the Bolognese. The English waxes were not only more realistic, but almost brutal, preferring anatomical accuracy to artistic flair. Robert Ballestriero (2010) describes:

> One of the major differences between the Italian and English wax models is the fact that the former are "alive" whilst the latter are "lifeless." The Florentine waxes are, moreover, irrespective of the subject, remarkably attractive; bodies seemed to be alive, pulsating; statues had a gentle look, a languid gaze; the "Venuses" had long hair left loose or gathered into seductive plaits and were often adorned by pearl necklaces ... the English waxes merely reproduced cadavers.

One of the nineteenth-century English modelers, Joseph Towne, had a very similar background to Susini: he had been trained from an early age in fine arts, had started to work as a wax modeler as a teenager, and had spent his entire fifty-year career perfecting his technique. Unlike Susini and the other modelers at La Specola, Towne found no reason to add any aesthetic embellishments to his work, which was intended exclusively for a medical audience. This audience was accustomed to authentic specimens, since cadavers were more readily available in England. Towne worked at Guy's Hospital and modeled some one thousand anatomical and pathological specimens after the dead to which he had access during his career. His models — which were carved from blocks of wax, rather than cast — are characterized (Ballestriero 2010) as practical and crude. Their pallor, livid flesh, and glazed eyes were true to death, and fashioned without any intent to soften the impression of being faced with a cadaver. Whether they were undergoing medical training or were completely uninitiated, viewers were faced with frozen grimaces locked in rigor mortis, with waxes that had no doubt been modeled on cadavers obtained chiefly from executed prisoners.

One of the Bolognese artists whose style and whose gender were atypical, was Anna Morandi Manzolini. Born in 1716, when Bologna was gaining fame as a research and teaching center for the natural sciences, she learned the art of wax modeling from her husband Giovanni Manzolini. They began working together in 1745, after he had finished an apprenticeship with a wax modeler, and together they studied both anatomy and its representation in wax. Morandi developed innovative dissection techniques so that she could more accurately visualize the human body and its parts. She translated what she saw into written descriptions and three-dimensional wax models. During her career, Morandi taught anatomy classes and demonstrated anatomy in her home. In 1755, the year she was widowed, she was recognized for her skill by Pope Benedict XIV, who awarded her a lifetime annual stipend. A member of the Academy of the Arts, which was part of the Institute of Science, she was given the title of the Chair of Anatomical Modeling at the University of Bologna in 1760. Unusually for the time, the university encouraged female academics, and she was one of several female professors at Bologna. As well as being in demand from the medical profession, she was also commissioned by private collectors across Europe to produce what they saw as artistic pieces (Panzanelli 2008). After Morandi died in 1774, her work—several examples of which remain—continued to influence anatomical studies by bringing together scientific and aesthetic qualities.

Clemente Susini was not the only modeler in wax to evoke artistic sensibilities in the presentation of human anatomy. He was also not the only artist to merit an honorary degree in human anatomy from working so closely with trained dissectors. The anatomical models of the eighteenth century exhibit "a troubling, sensual and surreal aspect, going well beyond the necessary scientific precision and the desired illusion," writes Lemire (1992), who goes on to describe them as "born from a close association between artists and anatomists—including some of the greatest in either field—and therefore located at the intersection of art and science" (Lemire 1992). But Susini was one of the most accomplished of the makers of anatomical waxes, held up as an example of a sculptor whose work is both didactic and evocative. The wax models prepared by Zumbo of the Bolognese school and England's Joseph Towne offered a sense of memento mori along with the graphic evidence of the cause of each demise. But Susini, of the Florentine school, brought his wax Venuses back to life.

Honoré Fragonard (1732–1799) and His Preparations

French anatomist Honoré Fragonard (1732–1799) made key contributions to the booming field of anatomical science which was still in many ways a social event at that time. "From the end of the sixteenth century, as science progressed and the social standing of the surgeon had risen, so too multiplied the activity of dissection. Not only the scholars, but a curious public too was keen to be initiated into the mysteries of the human body, and the spectacle of it was all the rage," writes Christophe Degueurce (2011). First, Fragonard began a career as a surgeon by apprenticing with a master surgeon in France and earning admission into France's Grasse Guild of Surgeons. After practicing for only three years, Fragonard was sought out and hired by Claude Bourgelat, who had founded the world's first veterinary school in Lyon. During his work as a demonstrator, Fragonard prepared a prototype of his famous specimen "Man on Horseback" by exposing and preserving the muscles of a horse and rider. While this wasn't one of them, he did bring a number of specimens with him in 1766 when he moved to Paris and then Alfort as professor of anatomy at the second veterinary school Bourgelat founded, this time at the initiation of the king.

The thousands of specimens that Fragonard prepared at the École nationale vétérinaire d'Alfort were placed on display in what came to be known as the school's cabinet du roi that was open to the public from the outset. He prepared specimens and skeletons of dozens of animals — especially the horse, but including llamas, sheep, monkeys, porpoises, and other diverse creatures. His surviving human écorchés, used in comparative anatomy at the veterinary school, include one bust with natural eyes and another with an open cranium. An existing full-body specimen known as "Man with Mandible" holds the jawbone of a horse and is outfitted with porcelain eyes. Other preparations that are assumed to be the work of Fragonard include a female body discovered in the attic of a hospital in 2000 and now curated at the Paris Institute of Forensic Medicine, the body of a young girl housed at the University of Montpellier 2, and a child's body auctioned by an antique dealer in 2004 and now in private hands. Fragonard preserved a number of human fetuses, including one holding its heart and another mounted on a donkey fetus, with reins and whips in hand. Still on display at Alfort is a fetus suspended by a thread that appears to be dancing and a group of three fetuses walking together on a base with their vascular systems highlighted and their crania opened.

To all who inquired about the collection, Fragonard replied, "Come and see." And they did, including German doctor Georg Ludwig Rumpelt, whose critical comment in 1779 could as easily have been directed at modern anatomist Gunther von Hagens' plastinates: "No preparation, even executed with the greatest care, holds to me any value if it does not demonstrate a new fact or the resolution of a debated issue. All their preparations, collected in the cabinet, satisfy only the gaze; few among them serve to demonstrate any new truths, to refute old errors; the refinements throughout are not instructive and demonstrate only the handiwork of their creator." But for von Hagens who pays him homage, and for the author Christophe Degueurce who curates his specimens, Fragonard was "an anatomist of genius, a practitioner unequalled" (2011).

Fragonard's pièce de résistance was the surviving "Horse and Rider." Though it's impossible to attribute some of the specimens to Fragonard with certainty, since he gave special training to his students who showed an aptitude for the work, this is not one of them. Fragonard was the subject of rumors at the time that he had used the body of a local grocer's daughter, but Degueurce (2011) points out that the span between her death and the unveiling of the specimen would not have allowed sufficient time for embalming. In addition — and perhaps more convincing, is the fact that the rider is male. The preparation was not intended to illustrate a horseman of the apocalypse, although the rider originally urged the horse on with reins and a whip. The props vanished in the 1950s, but "Horse and Rider" still stands.

The method Fragonard developed for producing his écorchés was to wash and shave the body, then open and drain the blood vessels. The temperature of the cadaver was raised by submerging it in successively warmer baths of water. He exposed the pulmonary artery and the aorta, and injected them first with a fine solution, then with a coarser one. The coronary arteries and heart required separate injections, and multiple injections were required for the veins. His injections included mutton tallow, pine resin, and essential oil. But rather than adding pigment to the solution, he painted the vessels afterward (arteries in red, veins in blue, nerves in white). Fragonard next removed the skin, isolating certain muscles and removing some of the organs for separate treatment. The bodies were selectively dissected to highlight specific systems: "mycologies" displayed the muscles, "angiologies" displayed the circulatory system, and "neurologies" displayed the nervous system. Fragonard wielded the scalpel with speed, so he could finish before decomposition set in. He desiccated the embalmed and anatomized body by submerging it in alcohol for as many as fifteen days, and then soaking it in vinegar spirit and corrosive sublimate. He painstakingly arranged the body on a frame, using thread, pads, and pins as necessary to achieve and maintain the desired position. Allowing the specimen to air-dry caused the muscles to shrink, so Fragonard would carefully reposition them. He reinflated or replaced the eyes. When set, the écorché was coated with varnish, which was sometimes pigmented to restore color to organs and muscles. Lastly, to ward off insects, he would apply coats of oil of turpentine.

Fragonard was successful with more than half of his preparations, which was considered very skilled given the difficulty of injecting cold cadavers with molten substances. He learned (and presumably taught) that the best bodies for écorchés were young (which ensured a flexible vascular system) and thin (which makes dissection of the fatty regions easier). But in addition to preparing écorchés, Fragonard was expert at producing what are known as corrosion casts. He made them by injecting the body's blood vessels with a corrosive-resistant material, then dissolving the surrounding tissues by submerging them in corrosive solution, and finally removing any remaining material by washing or delicate scraping. It was detail work like this to which Fragonard later referred when he argued the equality of the practitioner and the academic:

> That the professor is less knowledgeable than the anatomist is a fact in need of no proof. The one cannot do the work of the other just because he has been the other, and while the professor configures his own theoretical physiology based on that which he may or may not have seen, while he reads very eloquently from a text, it is undeniable that his faculties for learning are but stationary. Should it be his good fortune to forget nothing, still he remains at the point of educational advancement where he was ... when he quit the scalpel. The anatomist on the other hand, continually hunched over cadavers, advances in his research, realizes his conjectures; each day brings something new, for in anatomy we do not yet know everything; and like practical medicine, it cannot be learned from books [Degueurce 2011].

Fragonard's écorchés embody Vesalius' ideology of direct observation of the body over dogma and theory.

By investing them with gesture and emotion, Fragonard intended his écorchés to be artful. Apparently, Bourgelat didn't approve, and cut short his master embalmer's tenure at Alfort. Bourgelat dismissed Fragonard in 1771, calling him mad and claiming he didn't do his job. What's worse is that Bourgelat eradicated all credit to Fragonard for the specimens in the cabinet that he did prepare. Happily, Fragonard wasn't out of work for long, and his anatomical work continued uninterrupted. He prepared specimens for himself, but many times more for wealthy clients assembling their own cabinets, which had become all the rage. He was married and widowed within the space of three years, during and after which there are no historical records of Fragonard for more than a decade. It is known that he used some of his amassed wealth to purchase a large house from his cousin, Rococo painter Jean-Honoré Fragonard, in 1793, but it is unknown if he actually lived there.

What is known from the historical record is that Fragonard and two of his colleagues went before the national assembly in 1792 to propose the establishment of a national anatomy museum that would be the pride of France and comparable to Britain's Hunterian collection. They referred to it as a "temple of anatomy" not just because they hoped to house it in the Church of the Assumption. "Their ambition was to create ... a virtual cadaver factory, where a great number of specimens would be produced and sold, ensuring both the renewal of the collection and its continued financial support" (Degueurce 2011). The museum as envisioned would include an amphitheater, the specimens, a preparation laboratory, and lodgings for the employees. Believing that anatomists should be the curators of their own work, the three men hoped to take up annual appointments as director, inspector, and secretary/keeper of the cabinet, and would need to hire three anatomists, a custodian, and an assistant. Because of the difficulties he encountered in obtaining human cadavers for his specimens and the students at Alfort, the proposal included the provision that the principals of the museum be allowed to choose from the hospital those subjects that would be the most useful to them. If their plan were adopted, Fragonard was prepared to offer 1,500 specimens as the nucleus of the collection.

The proposal for a national museum was not acted on, but Fragonard was named to a commission established to inventory the anatomical cabinets across the country. In the national inventory of specimens gave each a number and label, and listing the preservation technique and condition. The total at Alfort was 3,033. Nearly a third of these — somewhere between 1,000 and 1,200 were transferred to Paris, where a world-renowned collection, now known as the Musée de Anatomie Delmas-Orfile-Rouvière or simply Musée Orfila, was assembled. Although now in storage, the collection of 5,500 objects included four specimens prepared by Fragonard, two of which (the mycology of monkey and the intestine of child) are still extant. In 1795, the Revolutionary government sought out and appointed Fragonard head of anatomy at the École de Santé de Paris (Paris School of Health). He was officially put in charge of directing research in anatomical preparation and training students in the art of injection. His appointment as "chief of anatomical works" by the board of public education allowed him a staff of six prosectors and the services of master anatomical model-maker André-Pierre Pinson.

At his death, Fragonard still worked at the Paris School of Health. At the end of his life, Fragonard was exhausted and had suffered financial losses, but his passion for anatomy remained as strong as ever. And the anatomical preparations he left behind are as popular as ever. As Degueurce points out (2011) there is today a resurgence of anatomy based

3. Anatomists as Preparators and Collectors (Honoré Fragonard)

on actual dissection. The pedagogical and spectacle coexist like they did in Fragonard's time. But time has distanced us from the work of the eighteenth-century anatomist, and while modern visitors are as prevalent as they were in the past, their relationship with the dead human body — long since co-opted by the medical profession — has noticeably modified our feelings about the écorchés. What were once teaching specimens are now museum pieces.

4

Anatomists as Superlatives and Showmen

The pages of England's *The Sussex Weekly Advertiser* from March/April 1790 relay the news of the execution and public dissection of fifty-year-old pedophile Richard Grazemark in March of that year. The man had many children by his daughter Jemima and "so violent was his unnatural passion for her, that he could not bear the thought of another possessing her." The day that she married, Grazemark burned down his house and attempted to kill his son-in-law with a knife. He was committed to Horsham Gaol, but was acquitted. He confessed afterward that he had stabbed his daughter to death in a field and "sat six hours on the body of the deceased and horrid to relate, in that situation, cut his own throat." When he recovered from the self-mutilation, he was sent to trial at Horsham for incest, murder, and attempted suicide, and was found guilty. At noon on the day of his execution, Grazemark was conveyed in a cart to the gallows, "which he approached without betraying the least mark of sorrow or contrition." Before he was hanged, he cried out, "Ladies and Gentlemen I wish you all well. I meant no harm." According to the contemporaneous account, he then "kicked off his slippers among the crowd and left the world exhibiting a most shocking instance of the depravity of human nature." It was further reported that his daughter had borne nine children by him over a period of fifteen years.

Grazemark's body was given over to surgeons Messrs. Price and Sopay for public dissection. Much of the crowd that had assembled to see the reviled man hang remained to see him dissembled. The anatomization was carried out on a platform set up for the purpose in the market square. The newspapers reported that "his skin which in some parts was a quarter of an inch thick was given to a tanner of that place for the purpose of manufacturing into leather, and several persons of Horsham have bespoken portions of it for soals [sic] to their shoes." The dissection revealed that the lanky and spare man had grown fat in prison, and perhaps was not the ideal subject for a lesson: "We do not hear that the young surgeons attempted to give lectures on the body but every one who chose to be present at the dissection was admitted whether led by curiosity or by the love of anatomy. In short the whole process was performed in public from the first incision to the boiling of the bones." The skeleton was presumably retained by one of the doctors, while the flesh was transported to the churchyard in baskets and buried. By that time the crowd would have dispersed, but would long remember what they had seen that day.

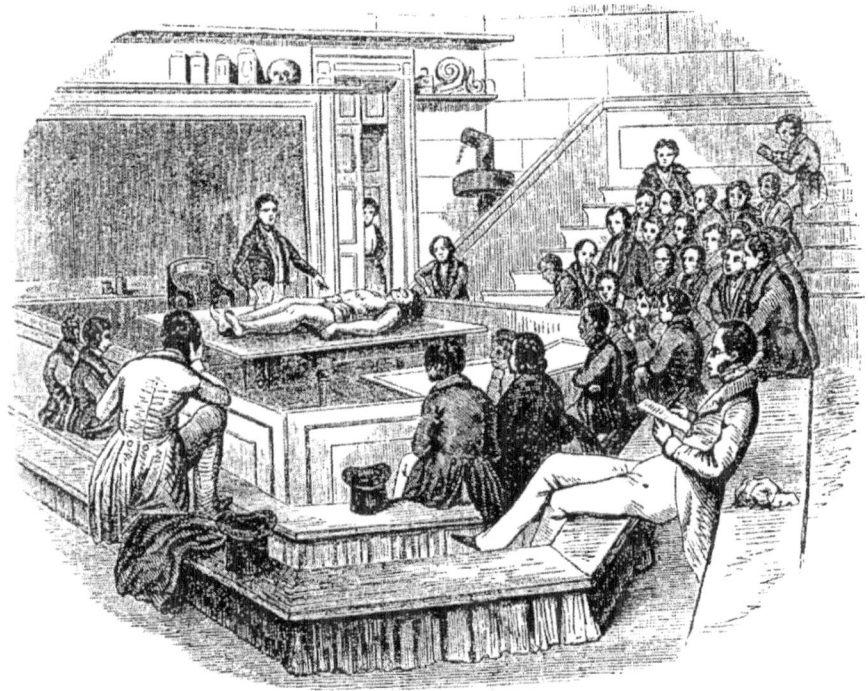

Male and female students in an anatomy class observe a dissection in an illustration from Henry Hollingsworth Smith's *Anatomical Atlas, Illustrative of the Structure of the Human Body*, published in Philadelphia in 1849 (*courtesy National Library of Medicine*).

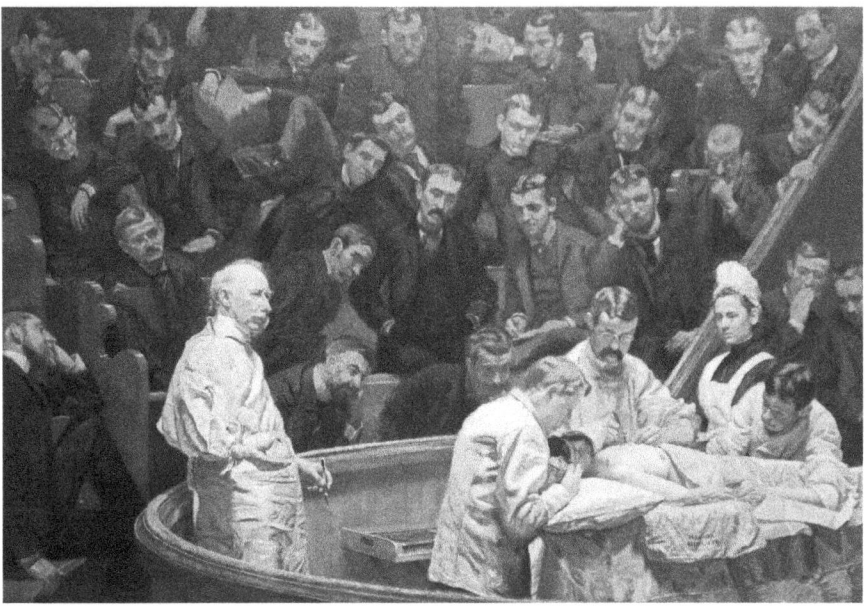

When professor of surgery Dr. D. Hayes Agnew announced his retirement, students from the University of Pennsylvania School of Medicine commissioned his portrait, "The Agnew Clinic." Philadelphia artist Thomas Eakins worked day and night to complete the painting in three months, so that it could be presented at the commencement ceremony on May 1, 1889. Eakins depicted the surgeon overseeing a surgery before a class of medical students. Although the subject of everyone's attention is a living patient rather than a cadaver, this example of scientific realism has been compared to Rembrandt's "The Anatomy Lesson of Dr. Nicolaes Tulp" and Hogarth's "The Reward of Crulty" (*courtesy University of Pennsylvania Art Collection, Philadelphia, Pennsylvania*).

Even when the motive for dissection is entirely didactic, when the setting is academic and off-limits to the public, it is still a performance. The professor takes a scalpel in hand — or uses a prepared prosection — to demonstrate what the medical students are expected to then carry out on the cadaver shared among them. At the turn of the century, the gross anatomy class was such a rite of passage that it became a mainstay of medical photography. In the ubiquitous dissection photographs that were taken at American medical schools, the images have often been restaged — to include all the members of a class, or to ensure that the exposure will have enough light. While appearing journalistic, these are well-planned images that capture — although not spontaneously — the dismantling of the human cadaver. In a student's scrapbook, the static photo conjured up the moving pictures of the event overseen by a necessarily proficient anatomist. A professor who was particularly charismatic or influential might be honored as the subject of a painting of him, his handiwork, and his audience — although this remained for the most part a seventeenth-century Dutch genre. Again, although it limits the viewer to a single glance at the staged event, and no opportunity to hear the concurrent narration, the canvas suggests what occurred before and after the sliver we see. We can imagine that the University of Pennsylvania medical students depicted observing a mastectomy in "The Agnew Clinic" were just as engaged and attentive while watching their first dissection by an instructor they will learn to emulate.

In the anatomical illustrations of the Renaissance, the anatomist is often missing from the scene. The cadaver is shown inviting, participating in, or even conducting its own anatomy demonstration. This self-dissection suggests the axiom "know thyself," while at the same time positioning the cadaver between the society of the living and the community of the dead. By being a willing accomplice to its own anatomization, the body symbolizes the power and truth of the study of this branch of human inquiry (Sawday 1995). In the poetry and literature of the late sixteenth and seventeenth centuries, the dissected body functioned as a source of meditation and instruction, reflected in art that echoes the iconography of the adoration of Christ's corpse, serves as a vanitas figure reminding readers of their own deaths, and represents mortality in contrast to the youthful students and mature professors in the illustrations of public dissection.

The early performance anatomical demonstration was influenced by medieval and Renaissance morality plays in which Death was one of the actors. As in the contemporary dramas of the day, the corpse was imagined alive by demonstrating how it functioned when living (Nunn 2005). Mirroring the journey of the moral tale leading to inevitable death, the fresh corpse was gradually reduced to a skeleton (van Dijck 2005). London's public interest in dissections influenced playwrights to feature the body, and public anatomies took on the characteristics of the staged dramas that had established their place in civic life. Actors and anatomists each performed to similar crowds in similar venues, though their shows served different purposes (Nunn 2005). Other similarities to theatrical performances included the division of the lessons into different phases, the institution of paid entrance tickets, the regulation of audience behavior, and the care taken over "production" (Ferrari 1987).

The anatomists had to actively consider their audiences. Like actors, the professors and dissectors on stage had to show their faces and clearly display the actions they performed (Ferrari 1987). Even though the body laying before them was the object of his action and the subject of his narrative, "the anatomist, rather than the cadaver, constituted the focal point of the anatomical theater" (van Dijck 2005). In describing the anatomy demonstrations of William Harvey, scholar Luke Wilson (1987) writes, "In the theater of anatomy, more than in the ordinary theater, to be a performer of oneself, an entertainer, has peculiar consequences. In gaining the spectator's complete attention, Harvey himself becomes, like the cadaver, a body 'subject to the view'— a body rather than simply an oral presence, because the performance *is* a performance and values enactment over information." It was Vesalius who began the trend in which the anatomist was the central performer on

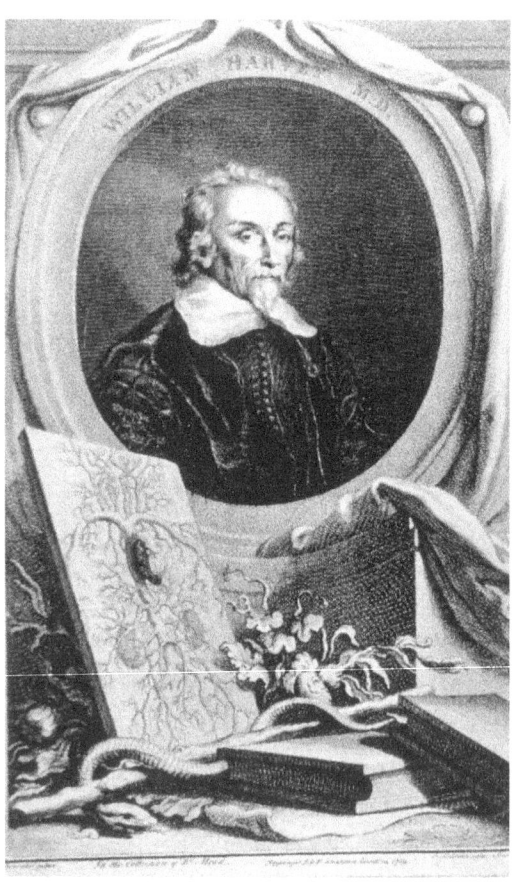

A 1732 engraving of English physician William Harvey by Jacobus Houbraken after a portrait by Wilhelm von Bemmel (*courtesy National Library of Medicine*).

the stage when he did away with the roles of demonstrator and ostensor, instead carrying out the functions himself—supposedly spontaneously and without reference to his notes (Wilson 1987).

From that point on, the anatomist was the star of the show, the impresario of this "early form of mass entertainment" (van Dijck 2005). He did not need to be cognizant of the many layers of meaning that the use of his skills raised. He did not need to be aware that through his dissection, he was transforming his subject from a particular corpse laid waste to a corpus of mental categories that make up the body of physiological knowledge (Wilson 1987). He could separate the rib cage and expose the internal organs without knowing that the formalized context of the dissections was necessary to counter their transgressive nature (Carlino 1999), or that carrying them out in a public setting ensured the legality and sanctity of the events (Wilson 1987). He could pursue the anatomization of the uterus, "an object sought after with an almost ferocious intensity in Renaissance anatomy theaters" (Sawday 1995), without understanding that the motivation for this was in mastering what was the source of all life—including his rational (male) intellect. Scholar Luke Wilson (1987) describes how the anatomist ritually dismantles the dead body, while his explanations of its functions symbolically reconstitute it. He characterizes the performance as a fantasy about the reversibility of mortality. This would have been more easily sensed by the Renaissance audience, who—amidst the ritual and memento mori in the anatomy theater—fully appreciated the symbolic significance of the corpse that the anatomist progressively disintegrated before them (Sawday 1995). But even a modern lay audience would not be ignorant of what the corpse on the table symbolizes: the eventual shared fate of all bodies.

No matter their rituals and traditions, their legal and punitive aspects, their theoretical underpinnings, or their didactic intentions, public dissections have always been valued as entertainment. They have been announced by engraved invitations and accompanied by music (Wetz 2004a). Reaching a height in sixteenth-century Italy, dissections were often accompanied by banquets, concerts, and theatrical performances, suggesting that they were understood as entertainment, of significance beyond their original medical context (Wilson 1987). When the barber-surgeons conducted their anatomy lectures, it was traditional to provide a lavish meal. The fact that the most important citizens turned out for dissections made them more social than scientific (Nunn 2005). Presumably, the audience members — who would have included nobility, clergy, faculty members, physicians, barbers, midwives, surgeons, apothecaries, artists, writers, scholars, and laypersons (Wetz 2004a) — were watching each other in addition to the anatomist and the body on the table. In fact, medical historian Michael Sappol (2002) says of early nineteenth-century America that fashionable men and women made appearances at anatomical theaters where they could observe *and be seen observing* anatomical dissections.

Over the centuries, the public dissection has only been instructive to a degree. The live event was the draw, specifically dissection of the dead body by the living anatomist who was so obviously familiar with it — or at least with butchering it. Not everyone in the anatomy theater had an unobstructed view, and lectures conducted in Latin were only understood by the initiated — although artists and others attended because they were fascinated by the combination of scientific aura, moral lesson, and morbid entertainment. The public anatomy lesson in the Renaissance, suggests author Jose van Dijck (2005), was most useful to the anatomist himself. It was of questionable use to students not already versed in prevailing anatomical theories, let alone to a general public. Because of its formality, the public demonstration did not bring about familiarity with the cadaver for either physicians or students. To be an effective teaching tool, it had to unite theoretical learning with practical ability, adds scholar Andrea Carlino (1999). It became apparent in the later seventeenth century, when a more detailed and scientific anatomical investigation was demanded, that a public anatomy was almost useless (Sawday 1995). Leading the lay viewer from observing a single dead body to abstract theories about living bodies (van Dijck 2005) was a tall order, made easier by the interested "scientific gentlemen" of the early 1800s, who craved the rare and modern experience of being present at a dissection (Sappol 2002). The goal of disseminating knowledge to the average viewer was achieved to some extent in later nineteenth-century America, when learning anatomy was connected to taking care of one's health: "In the Antebellum period, anatomy overflowed the boundaries of professional medical discourse and performance, and became important to the American middle class" (Sappol 2002). Just as European students had done centuries earlier, the American public at that time flocked to anatomy lectures, whether or not they featured an actual dissection.

"Anatomical performances signified a bold and contentious appropriation of the body and of death," states Sappol (2002). Describing the anatomical theater of Bologna in its heyday, scholar Giovanna Ferrari (1987) writes, "The anatomist presented himself as the depository of the secrets of the microcosm, and the possessor of an intellectual form of knowledge rather than of a practical and therapeutic one. The original didactic purpose of the anatomical investigations now seemed almost irrelevant..." (Ferrari 1987). It was by attending anatomy demonstrations that artists could more accurately represent the human figure and that young men could legitimately gaze at a nude female form. A multitude of meanings and motivations hovered over the early anatomists, who defied superstition and taboos about the dead in the pursuit of knowledge. The barber-surgeons, by delivering the second half of a legal sentence, allowed criminals to expiate their wrongdoing by giving over their bodies to the benefit of the common good. The professors who unrolled ancient Egyptian mummies in Victorian lecture halls to both excited and edified awed crowds. And today's celebrity anatomist Gunther von Hagens patterns himself on the past as he presents dissection as a postmodern entertainment.

Public dissections were rare enough in the fourteenth and fifteenth centuries that no auditorium was necessary. Dissectors performed outdoors on windy sites that would carry away any unpleasant odors, or accommodated observers in makeshift rooms. Vacant churches and the chapels of former monasteries — San Francesco in Bologna, the Church of St. Elizabeth in Basel, and St. Jacob's chapel in Tübingen — were utilized for the purpose (Wetz 2004a). And sometimes temporary anatomical theaters were constructed for an annual event and dismantled afterward. Based on ancient Roman amphitheaters, the temporary wooden theaters were lit by torches and staffed with an usher and guards (to assist and, if necessary, restrain the eager crowds), and a steward (to collect the admission fee, which was distributed to the poor for the salvation of the dissected cadaver, after all expenses were recovered). The public dissection followed a particular protocol, and guests were seated in the temporary structures according to rank. In Italian universities, the audience was limited to teaching faculty and students who had been matriculated for at least one year. A body of either gender was provided by the rector per the civil authorities, with the medical students officiating and the doctors free to discuss the structures that had been or would be dissected (French 1999).

It was in Italy that the university community first responded to the need for a permanent anatomical theater for the regular performances of the anatomists. Alexander Benedictus designed a theater for Padua in 1497 with the following considerations in mind: sufficient seating with good visibility for a large audience, a well-lit central dissection table, adequate ventilation, and places to post the guards and stewards. A cen-

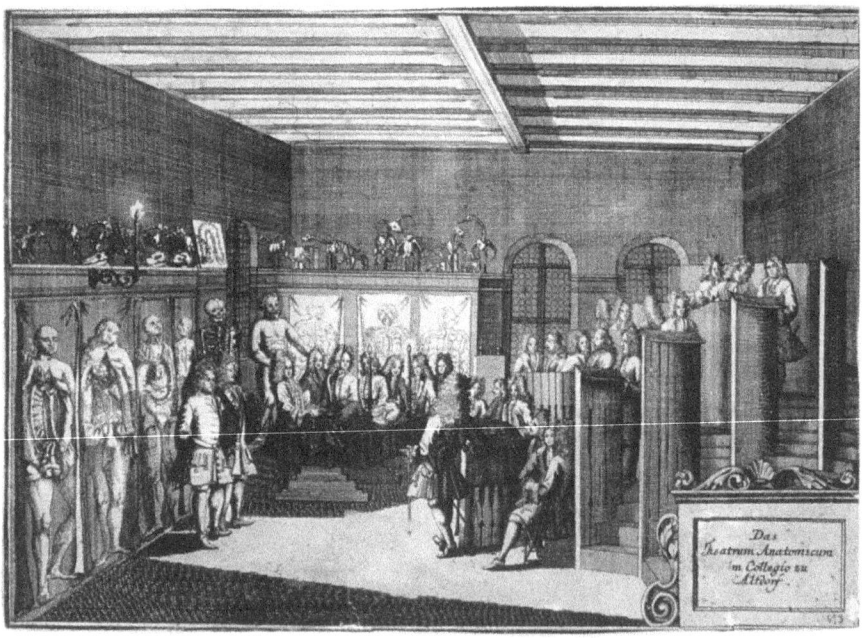

The interior of an anatomical theater at a German college circa 1650, illuminated by candlelight, is shown here. The demonstration is being observed by a number of students. Large-scale anatomical charts are pinned to the walls and small skeletons are arranged on a shelf (*courtesy National Library of Medicine*).

tury later, in 1594, Fabricius ab Aquapendente planned a permanent theater to be incorporated into an existing building at the University of Padua. It rises through two stories of the campus centerpiece, Bo Palace, and its construction was aided by the local skill in shipbuilding. The design served as a model for anatomical theaters that followed in Leiden (1597), Copenhagen (1643), Altdorf (1650), Groningen (1655), Uppsala (1662), Amsterdam (1691), Berlin (1720), and Halle (1727).

The wooden, funnel-shaped structure of the Padua theater had both pros and cons. The six concentric rings separated by balustrades allowed for a large number of visitors, but with no seating. The rector, professors, nobles, dignitaries, and members of the medical college occupied the front row; students stood in the second and third rows; and the remaining rows were open to the public. The dissection table at the center of the well could be lowered hastily through a trapdoor if necessary (not a tunnel, as is popularly believed), but this left little floor space for the lecturer, his assistants, and the eight students required to hold candles to illuminate the demonstration due to the lack of natural light (Schumacher 2007). Official dissections were held at the Padua theater, but the events did not keep pace with the academic need, so anatomies held unofficial dissections for smaller audiences in pharmacies or professors' homes (Malomo et al. 2006). Nevertheless, the formal theater was in use for nearly three centuries and — because of its prototypical design and the renown of the men who lectured there — has been preserved to this day. The anatomy theater at Padua is now a museum, adorned with the skulls of noted professors exhumed by phrenologists in the nineteenth century, and is open for guided tours.

Unlike the circular theater that originated in Padua, the anatomical theater in Bologna built the following year (1595) followed a rectangular style that stemmed from the design of medieval meeting-places. Because of the timing of the annual dissections, the theater was decorated to match the ceremonial and celebratory aspects of the event. For over 150 years, a public dissection was held to coincide with the annual carnival, a time when the university was on vacation, the weather was cold, and transgressive things were permitted (Carlino 1999). The event was neither a theoretical anatomy lesson, nor a dissection performed by a teacher for the instruction of his students, but a complex ceremony, unique because of its ritualized features and its survival over time (Ferrari 1987). The Bologna theater was magnificently decorated for the occasion, with damask hung on the wood-paneled walls, candlesticks illuminating the room, and two waxen torches lighting the head and foot of the table. In lateral niches stood statues of the fathers of medicine — Hippocrates, Galen, and Mondino de Liuzzi — and the university's most famous anatomy professors. Above them rested twenty busts of the college's founder and faculty members. The canopy was supported by two wooden statues of human anatomy (Ferrari 1987). All in all, an awe-inspiring setting for the anatomists to take the stage.

The first lesson of the two-week event was well-promoted. Public notices were posted in Latin indicating the date and time of the inaugural lesson, which — like the final lesson — was attended by the most eminent city officials. The cadaver lay for ten to fifteen days in the middle of the theater as a series of medical, philosophical, and anatomical lectors presided over its dissection. Each morning and afternoon began with a general introductory lesson and was organized around a particular organ or system. In order of their precedence, the scholars in that subject spoke and initiated a discussion among the audience by posing questions. Afterward, the anatomy professor demonstrated his lesson directly from the cadaver, which had been prepared in advance by the dissector. An average of sixteen to twenty topics, and in some years thirty or more, were covered. During this time, masses paid for by the professor were said for the souls of those dissected (Ferrari 1987).

Despite the decorum of proceedings, it was apparently difficult to control the rowdy crowd of several hundred. Disturbances might be caused by family and friends objecting to a dissection, unruly spectators, barber-surgeons protesting fees, or dignitaries questioning their seating assignments (Carlino 1999). Laws were enacted in the seventeenth century forbidding chatting, laughing, asking indecent questions, and grabbing organs from the dissector (Nunn 2005) even though the dissecting table was protected from the crowd by a balustrade. Nevertheless, the formal seating arrangement was maintained. The prior and counselors sat on benches at one end and the authorities at the other. Along the side walls to the right sat members of the university community, its porters, and the notary. To the left sat the doctors, arranged by seniority and surrounded by the students. Ordinary citizens were admitted, but relegated to leftover seats or standing room. And for those who wanted to see without being seen, the anatomy theater of Bologna had a secret compartment from which "authorities, ladies or other persons" could view the dissection. Like the Padua theater, the theater in Bologna is now a museum.

Rather than waiting until it was abandoned for demonstrations, the anatomy theater built in Leiden, Holland, in 1597 was converted to an anatomical museum during the times it was not in use for the dissections carried out centuries ago. It was modeled on the theater at Padua, but was slightly larger and had six wide ascending rows of seats that did not block the illumination from the large windows. The Leiden theater had been built in a former church, and the moral lessons suffused the anatomy demonstrations, as was typical of the time. Its interior was decorated with the skeletons of animals and humans, all of which had been dissected within, and the walls were painted with mottoes about death and repentance: "Nascentes morimur" ("To be born is to die"), "Mors ultima linea rerum" ("Death is the line that marks the end of all"), "Mors sceptra ligonibus aeqvat" ("Death wrenches from the hand the scepter as well as the spade"), and "Pulvis & umbra sumis" ("We are dust and shadow"). Begun under the administration of Dr. Pieter Pauw, the decorative arrangement of the collection of anatomical skeletons and preparations at Leiden set a precedent for such displays in Holland and the rest of Europe that continued throughout the eighteenth century (Hansen 1996). Once it became internationally renowned and heavily visited, an engraving of the theater — complete with memento mori messages — was prepared in 1610 and sold to tourists. Later, beginning in 1671, a series of guidebooks was offered. An edition published in English in 1727 was entitled *A Catalogue of all the Chiefest rarities in the Publick Theater and Anatomie Hall*. The guidebook described the anatomical exhibits with an emphasis on the moralistic message. It noted that one skeleton was that of a woman who had committed suicide, and the bones of two others were mothers who had killed their children. A caption noted "Catherine of Hamburg, strangled for theft" and pointed out that the man astride the skeleton of an ox had been executed for stealing cattle. Hanson (1996) explains, "By displaying the skeletons of criminals whose cadavers had been dissected in the theaters, the university doctors were justifying the use of bodies for a purpose beyond the temporal limitations of the civic execution and the public anatomy lesson. The bodily remains of these malefactors, instead of being dissected and buried, were transformed into eloquent displays in the form of vanitas-inspired art for the edification of the Leiden community." The lessons were learned by the locals and by patrons from afar.

Sightseers were plenty, as no cultured late sixteenth- or early seventeenth-century English traveler would neglect to visit the anatomy theaters at Leiden, Bologna, or Padua (Sawday 1995). When dissections were not in session, they were treated to the sight of anatomical rarities collected by the university's professors, art and artifacts that were displayed on the walls, and scientific instruments that were of more historical than practical value. A dissection could, in a sense, be prolonged indefinitely by retaining, preparing, and displaying in the theater the skeletons and organs of the cadavers that had been opened within its halls. "This was especially true in the cases of dissected criminals, whose skeletal remains or prepared body parts served the additional moralizing function of reminding the audience of the consequences of vice and antisocial behavior" (Hansen 1996). The anatomy theater designed by Inigo Jones for London's barber-surgeons (erected in 1638 and demolished in 1784) had its own notable exhibits: a pair of male and female human skins, a mummy skull, and the skeletons of executed subjects. It drew a curious Samuel Pepys to attend the dissection of a seaman hanged for robbery in 1662, after which the diarist noted that he ate a fine dinner and returned with Dr. Scarborough to see the body alone (Sawday 1995).

The building of anatomy theaters had mushroomed in England and abroad during the seventeenth century. The "Domus anatómica" in Copenhagen was based on the Leiden model, but anatomist Simon Paulli added a rotating dissection table, which could be turned in the direction of the sun. But the ongoing problem of illumination was solved in Uppsala. The placement of the anatomical theater on the top floor of the existing main building of the university — the "Gustavianum" — allowed a cupola to be added to the roof, through which natural light could beam down (Schumacher 2007). Not only was the sunlight practical, it had the effect of turning the theater into a "shrine" to anatomy. The anatomy theater was in general viewed as a sort of sacred stage. It was — like a temple or church — to be beautifully proportioned like the human body. It was visually spectacular and in construction emulated the judicial court, dramatic stage, and religious basilica. Following a carnivalesque public execution, the dissection within struggled to transcend the spectacle of disorder and assert order and harmony through a ritual of investigation. The addition of memento mori symbols made the anatomy theater an architectural lesson in human mortality (Sawday 1995).

By the eighteenth century, nearly every medical school had its own anatomical theater (Wetz 2004a). Not only was the edifice important to the university in attracting students, it was an important milestone in the growth of a city. Author Jonathan Sawday (1995) explains, "The anatomy theatre was a register of civic importance, an index of the intellectual advancement of a community, an advertisement of a city's flourishing cultural and artistic life." The progress in anatomy and an increase in the number of students brought changes by the eighteenth century. Anatomical theaters stood on their own, and were built with optimal acoustics and visibility for a large-capacity crowd. With the 1694 anatomical theater of the Academy of Surgeons in Paris as a precursor, the Grand Amphitheatre des Ecoles de Chirurgie was erected in the same city between 1768 and 1775. Light poured in from the ceiling and the semicircular seating arrangement — modeled after the Roman Pantheon — accommodated an audience of 1,400.

Improvements in embalming led to a wider incorporation of the corpse in the anatomical curriculum and prompted the need not just for theaters, but for entire anatomical institutes with separate rooms for the preparation and storage of cadavers, display of specimens, and laboratory and research work. Two types of buildings arose. The Senckenberg Institute of Anatomy, built between 1768 and 1776 in Frankfurt, Germany, with a central auditorium and two symmetrical wings, served as the model for anatomical institutes in Dorpat (1827) and Erlangen (1826–27). The drawbacks of this configuration, which did not facilitate communication and transfer between rooms, was overcome with an anatomist-designed rectangular building that had an extended auditorium in front with semi-circular rows of seats and ample lighting and ventilation. This was the layout adopted in Munich (1826), Gottingen (1828–29) and Greifswald (1854–55) (Schumacher 2007).

Subsequent anatomical buildings followed two styles, but had common characteristics. Whether aligned (typical of Europe) or grouped (typical of England), the rooms allowed continuous access without the theater being a barrier between them. At the same time, they maintained strict separation between the lecture hall and the rooms designated as dissecting halls, laboratories, and museums. Neither of these types of anatomical institutes were typical of the U.S., where anatomy rooms were incorporated into large biomedical complexes and theaters were no longer based on the traditional anatomical theater, but were instead modeled after the movie theater (Schumacher 2007). Once anatomy became more than descriptive — and each of the applied sciences like cell biology, embryology, and neurology required specialized equipment and laboratories of their own — the anatomical theater became less central physically and theoretically, and dissection became less of a performance. Nevertheless, the anatomist still held center stage with the cadaver.

Nicolaes Tulp (1593–1674) and His Fame

Even if you don't know much about the career of Dutch anatomist Nicolaes Tulp, you no doubt recognize him from what is perhaps the most well-known dissection scene: "Anatomy Lesson of Dr. Nicolaes Tulp" (1632) by Dutch artist Rembrandt van Rijn (1606–1669). Leiden-educated physician and surgeon Dr. Tulp had been appointed as lecturer of the Surgeon's Guild in 1628. He is depicted explaining the musculature of the arm with reference to an anatomy textbook (possibly the famous *De Humani Corporis Fabrica* by Andreas Vesalius) and without the inclusion of the many surgical instruments he would have used to perform the actual dissection. The oil painting marks a historical event — Dr. Tulp's second public dissection on January 31, 1632. The subject, Leiden resident Adriaan "Aris Kindt" ("Aris the Kid") Adriaanszoon, had just been hanged after being convicted of armed robbery for stealing a coat. (He had begun his criminal career, which included the attempted murder of a well-to-do citizen, nine years earlier.) Adriaanszoon was dissected in Leiden's anatomical theater, but most of the spectators are excluded

4. Anatomists as Superlatives and Showmen (Nicolaes Tulp)

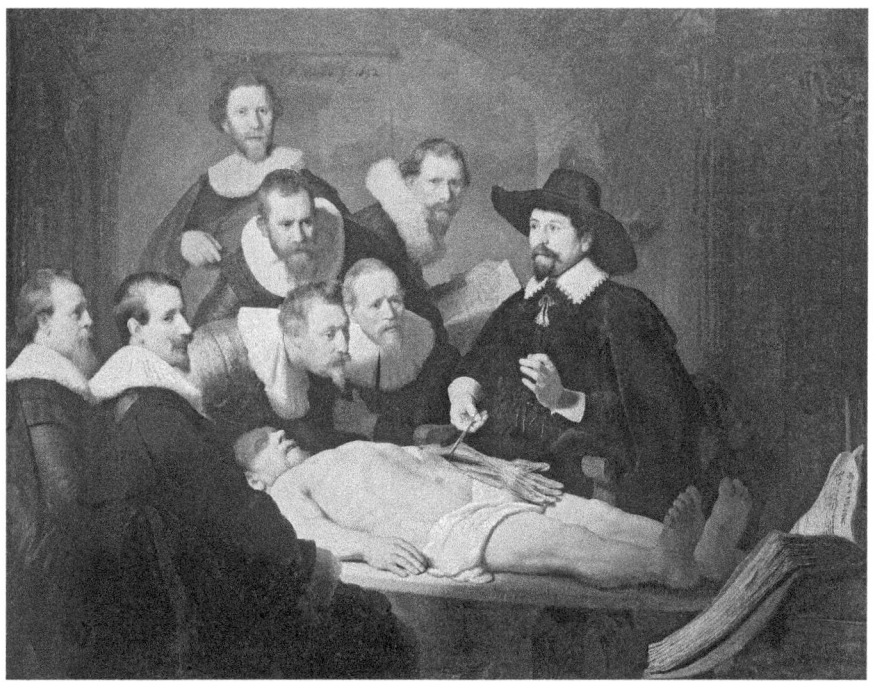

"The Anatomy Lesson of Dr. Nicolaes Tulp," a 1632 group portrait by Dutch master Rembrandt van Rijn, depicts the public dissection of a hanged criminal by the Leiden-educated surgeon who had been appointed as lecturer by the Amsterdam Surgeon's Guild four years earlier. The dissection was performed in Leiden's anatomical theater, but instead of including the audience of townspeople, Rembrandt was paid to include surgeons who may or may not have been present. He also employs artistic license by depicting the anatomization of an extremity before the rest of the body had been dissected (*Royal Picture Gallery Mauritshuis, The Hague*).

from the canvas. Instead, the innovative lighting and composition of the painting, and the intense gazes of the grouped men, make it clear that the observers outside the painting make up that audience of townspeople. But Rembrandt — whose reputation climbed quickly after the commission — employs artistic license by painting in surgeons who paid to be included and may not have been present at the dissection. He also strays from reality by showing the dissection of the lower arm while the rest of the body remains intact, when in fact the rest of the body would already have been dissected and virtually unrecognizable by the time the forearm was anatomized (Sawday 1995). The painting is therefore an idealized group portrait rather than a record of the event.

The same liberty was taken by Rembrandt in his later painting "The Anatomy Lesson of Dr. Joan Deyman" (1656). Although only a fragment survives, the canvas depicts eight figures and Tulp's successor dissecting the brain of Juris Fontaine, a criminal executed in January 1656. Originally hung in the Guild Room of Amsterdam Surgeon's Hall, the painting contradicts the fact that the dissection of the thorax would have preceded the probing of the brain (Sawday 1995). In the first painting of this genre, "The Osteology Lesson of Dr. Sebastiaen Egbertsz" (1619) by Nicolaes Elias Pickenoy, the curious onlookers who paid admission to be present at the event — the annual public dissection carried out by the Dutch Surgeon's Guild — have been omitted from the painted scene, which shows only the members of the guild gathered around the skeleton with Dr. Egbertsz poised over it. Nine such paintings of the annual dissection commissioned to hang in the Guild Room have survived to the present day. More dramatic than informative about the dissection, the anatomy theater, and the paying audience, we can assume Dr. Tulp was pleased with his depiction.

In fact, Dr. Nicolaes Tulp was himself a showman. When still a student, he changed his name from the very common Claes Pieterszoon to the more scholarly Nicolaus Petreius. Once he had established his Amsterdam practice, he changed his name again. This time, in a nod to the city's love of tulips, he called himself Nicolaes *Tulp* (the Dutch word for tulip). He used a coat-of-arms in the form of a red tulip to decorate his house and coach, and later to stamp official documents during his three terms as mayor of Amsterdam. Perhaps most tellingly, Dr. Tulp patterns himself after Vesalius, who is shown dissecting a forearm and hand in the frontispiece of history's most famous medical textbook, possibly to be seen as his successor.

Georges Cuvier (1769–1832) and His Venus

Georges Cuvier is one of the most famous names in science. The French naturalist and zoologist was a principal founder of the fields of paleontology and comparative zoology, and he established the facts of extinction. He did not, however, believe in evolution, and he espoused the racist views of the craniologists of the nineteenth century. After Cuvier's death, his own brain was examined by his scientific colleagues and — weighing in at more than four hundred grams above average — used to bolster their theories of the superiority of the white race. During his life, Cuvier had the opportunity to examine a well-known "specimen" of what the craniologists considered the most inferior race, but it wasn't her skull or its contents that excited his interest.

Famous for her prominent buttocks and her genital apron, the woman known as the "Hottentot Venus" was compelled to disrobe and pose for the scientific illustrations of several famous naturalists who came to see her in Paris. The public had a less clinical view of her in Piccadilly Circus, where — exhibited in a cage — she offered her backside up to be pinched, but kept her private treasure to herself. The woman's name was Saartjie Bjartmaan, she was twenty years old, and she had come from Capetown, South Africa, in 1810, with the permission of the governor. To scientists, she was proof of evolution; to her public audience, she was a curiosity; but to abolitionists, she was a cause, having been born into slavery and — although she had denied it in a Dutch court — exhibited

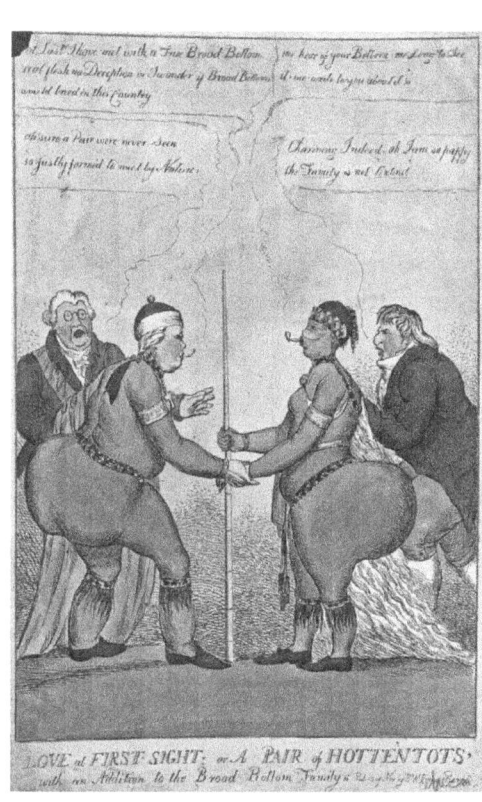

"Hottentot Venus," an early 18th-century etching of "living specimen" Saartjie Baartman and a fellow Khoisan countrywoman, standing with a pole between them and pipes in their mouths. The men flanking them are astounded by their large buttocks and hoping for a look at their elongated labia (*Wellcome Images*).

against her will. She has become an icon in her home country, where "Hottentot" is now a pejorative term replaced by "Khoi-Khoi." Her case became more prominent when an account was published by American scientist Stephen Jay Gould.

As a young woman, Saartjie had been taken into the custody of free black Pieter Cesars, a hunter and trader, who brought her to the Capetown home of his brother Hendrik and wife to be a live-in wetnurse to their daughter. Hendrik worked for British Army medical officer Alexander Dunlop. Saartjie's relationship with a drummer was encouraged and she got pregnant in 1807, which allowed her to nurse her own baby and that of her employers (Holmes 2007). But her baby, the name and gender of which is not known, died before the age of two. Dunlop, who had fallen out of favor with his superiors and was expected to return to England to await a new post, convinced Pieter and Hendrik that Saartjie — though unremarkable among her own people — had lucrative potential as a scientific curiosity in England. The men conspired to take her to England and option the rights to her exhibition on a contract basis.

Saartjie was apparently smuggled out of South Africa as a stowaway on a vessel destined for England in Spring of 1810. She had an understanding with Dunlop and Cesars that they would send her back to Cape Town, at their expense and with all her earnings, after six years. She was charged with devising an engaging routine that she would have the stamina to repeat for the four hours a day, six hours a week, that she would be on stage. In addition to her daytime public appearances, she also gave private evening viewings to parties of twelve who booked in advance. A one-piece, form-fitting body stocking made it appear that she wore little clothing, and this notion was enhanced by concealing any seams, buttons, and hooks in the publicity images (Holmes 2007).

Since slavery was unconstitutional in Britain, Saartjie's confinement was challenged in court and she became the cause of abolitionists who believed she was compelled to exhibit herself and did not do so of her own free will. Hearing Saartjie testify that she had given her consent and had no desire to return to Africa prior to the six-year term of her agreement, which she produced, the judge declined to prosecute and instead cautioned Dunlop and Cesars, and recommended further action if there were grounds for public indecency (Holmes 2007). Saartjie's supporters found her display degrading to her state of "noble savagery" and believed she was being exploited sexually and scientifically. But the trial merely ensured the exhibition's continued success. Following her display in Piccadilly, she toured England in 1811, appearing in Brighton and Bath, and Ireland the following year, with a five-day performance in Limerick. In 1814, she arrived in France and was soon the center of the debate about race between eminent scientists Georges Cuvier and Étienne Geoffroy Saint-Hilaire of the Musée National d'Histoire Naturelle.

In Paris, Saartjie performed from noon till six, then spent her evenings at restaurants, cafes, and bars drumming up further business, or at private parties, dinners, or salons being ogled by members of "polite society." Dunlop had died of unknown causes in 1812, so Cesars extended the hours of Sartjie's daily performance from six to ten hours to maximize profits, since his six-year stake was coming to an end. Sartjie's health began to suffer, and exhaustion, recurrent bouts of flu, and the effects of her heavy drinking took their toll. While she was offstage in her sickbed, Cesars took up the offer of a showman named Réaux to manage the Hottentot Venus exhibition and returned to Cape Town. Réaux soon had Saartjie up and working a twelve-hour shift. And with his complicity — because he could use their report as further credential for her exhibition — Saartjie was summoned by police to appear before a panel of academicians headed by Cuvier, Saint-Hilaire, and Henri de Blainville for examination. Before the group of zoologists, naturalists, anatomists, physiologists, and artists at the Jardin du Roi, Saartjie stood on a platform as they studied and sketched her over a period of several days. Against her strong objections, Cuvier succeeded in convincing her to remove her clothes, but she used a handkerchief to cover her modesty. Deprived of the view of the legendary "apron," de Blainville simply drew what he imagined it looked like, and this cartouche of her sex organs and their supposed wing-like elongation appeared in a scholarly journal in 1816 (Holmes 2007).

Saartjie never fully recovered from her illness of the winter of 1814. The scientists who had examined her made discreet offers to Reaux to pay a sum of money upon delivery of her corpse for the purpose of anatomical dissection. Ironically, the *eau de vie*— brandy — that warmed her body and spirit was the same liquid that the scientists at the Musée used to prepare their specimens. She did not keep body and soul together much longer, dying on December 29, 1815. Instead of reporting the death to the authorities, Reaux contacted Saint-Hilaire in person. Saint-Hilaire notified the mayor of Saartjie's death and his intention to remove her body to the anatomy laboratories "in the interests of the progress of human knowledge" (Holmes 2007). He also wrote to the prefect of police to request permission to do so at the Musée, even though legal dissection was only authorized at the University of Paris and the Petie Hospital, after which the remains were supposed to be buried at Clamart Cemetery. Permission was granted under the condition that Saint-Hilaire take measures to preserve decency and coordinate with the police to make an official record of the handover of the body.

Less than twenty-four hours after her death, Saartje's body was delivered to the Musée with two documents: her contract with Dunlop and her birth certificate. She lay naked on her back on Cuvier's anatomy bench. As the dissection was being performed, the *Annales Politiques, Morales et Littéraires* reported that it would "provide M. Cuvier with an extremely curious chapter for his account of the varieties of the human species" (Holmes 2007). He later extrapolated from the small size of her skull that she lacked intelligence, while at the same time noting that she was fluent in three languages and had an excellent memory. Assistants helped at the table, cleared blood, and mixed the necessary solutions: lard, plant oil, and Chinese wax for making plaster casts of her body, internal organs, and external genitalia; distilled alcohol for the fluid preservation of her brain and sexual organs; and potassium hydroxide (caustic potash) for the boiling of her bones (Holmes 2007). Cuvier himself conducted a full dissection, removing and preserving her brain and genitals. As he published in the *Memoires du Muséum d'Histoire Naturelle* two years after the dissection, Cuvier confirmed that the protuberance of her buttocks was due to fat. And not only did he relish in solving the mystery of her apron (it was a 3–4" labia minora), he preserved it. The note that accompanied the specimen read, "I have the honor to present to the academy the genital organs of this woman prepared in a manner that leaves no doubt about the nature of her [apron]." He then ordered the laboratory cleaned and supervised the disarticulation and boiling of Saartjie's skeleton.

4. Anatomists as Superlatives and Showmen (Georges Cuvier)

Obituaries announced that the Hottentot Venus had died of smallpox, although the cause diagnosed by Cuvier as "eruptive and imflammatory disease" could as easily have been pleurisy, syphilis, or pneumonia — especially in combination with her alcoholism. Saartjie's death mask shows her face to have been painfully swollen. After the dissection — and until his own death in 1832, Cuvier displayed the jars containing Saartjie's brain and genitals just outside the door to his private apartments at the Musée in his Cabinet d'Anatomie Comparée. They were, as described in 1822, preserved in bottles of greenish glass without any mode of suspension (Holmes 2007). Her skeleton also joined the forty-one other human skeletons in the gallery, including those of eleven other Hottentots. Later, the specimens — along with the cast of Saartjie's corpse — were put on public display, where they remained until 1974.

More than 150 years after her dissection, Saartjie's preserved genitals were rediscovered in a storage area alongside the brains of illustrious nineteenth-century scientists including Cuvier, whose body had also been dissected per his own precise instructions. Coincident with the end of apartheid in 1994, South Africa president Nelson Mandela formally requested repatriation of Saarjie's remains of French president François Mitterrand. After much negotiation and the misinformation that the remains had been accidentally destroyed in the early 1980s (Holmes 2007), the French government handed over the remains in a ceremony held at the South African embassy in Paris in April 2002. They were specially crated and flown to Johannesburg three days later. In August, after Khoisan rituals were performed, a state funeral was held and Saartjie was buried in a casket decorated with aloe wreaths in the rural town of Hankey on a hill overlooking the Gamtoos River Valley, near where she had grown up.

In her essay in *The Gendered Cyborg*, Linda Schiebinger faults Cuvier for his obsession with Bjartmaan's genitalia. African American women had already been stereotyped as promiscuous, so scientific studies about them predictably focused on their sexuality. Much had been written and speculated about the "Hottentot apron," also called the "veil of shame" or the "drape of decency." Because few Europeans had seen this characteristic, which they viewed as a deformity, they argued about its very existence. By the time Cuvier performed his dissection, interest in the apron had reached voyeuristic proportions and he claimed that his examination answered the most celebrated question in natural history. Scheibinger relates that Cuvier's descriptions of Bjartmaan's physique were bestial throughout and that more than half of his report focused in her genitals, breasts, buttocks, and pelvis. By virtue of her gender and her race, she was nothing more than a sexual animal, underlined by the fact that her skin was removed, prepared, and put on display in England, and her labia was consigned to a jar in France.

Thomas Pettigrew (1791–1865) and His Mummies

In the nineteenth century, during the height of Egyptomania, it was quite fashionable among the upper classes to invite one's friends to an "unrolling" if you had an ancient Egyptian mummy in your collection of antiquities. Invitations would be engraved and sent, and the small crowd would assemble around a table on which the wrapped body lay. Its secrets would be revealed by the host, who would remove the outer and inner wrappings and any amulets they contained, revealing the body of the ancient Egyptian. The procedure has been described as voyeuristic, even though the body itself was often not opened by "armchair archaeologists." Instead, it was at that point usually donated to a museum, especially after the publication of fictional accounts of mummies by Edgar Allan Poe, Sir Arthur Conan Doyle, and others introduced the idea that they would bring bad luck to the households in which they were kept.

The unwrapping of a mummy was a social, rather than a scientific occasion, and it was meant to impress. One of the earliest mummy unrollings was carried out by French consul in Cairo Benoît de Maillet (1656–1738), who unwrapped a mummy to delight a group of French tourists in 1698. But even when unrollings *were* intended as a scientific pursuit, proper procedure was thwarted. An apothecary named C. Hertzog undertook the unwrapping and description of an ancient Egyptian mummy in 1718, but did not conserve the remains and instead ground them up in a powder — as was the practice of the time — to be sold as

4. Anatomists as Superlatives and Showmen (Thomas Pettigrew)

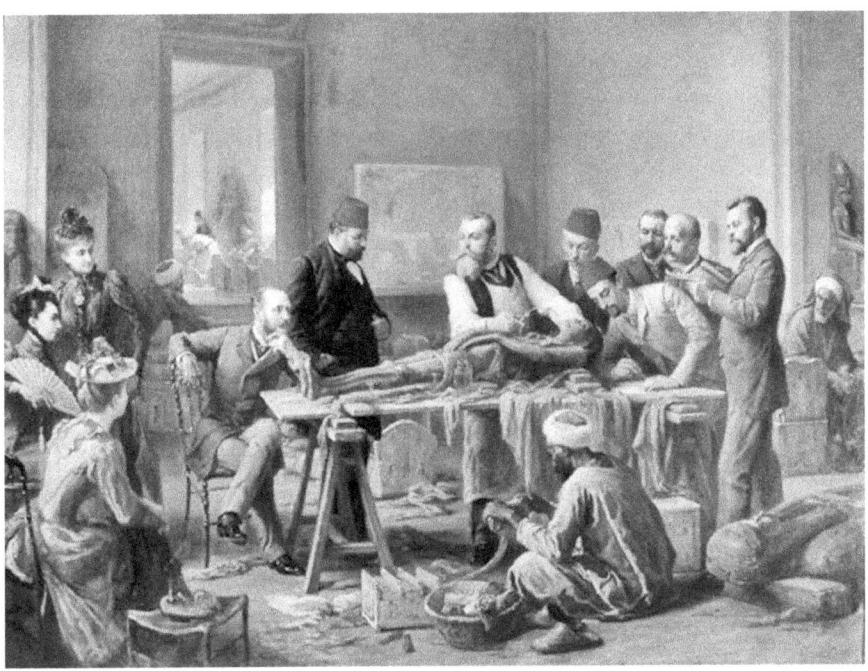

In the late 19th century French artist Paul Dominique Philippoteaux was commissioned to paint "Examination of the mummy of the Priestess of Ammon," depicting the unwrapping of ancient Egyptian priestess Ta-udjat-Ra, whose 21st Dynasty mummy was found with others in the Deir El Bahri cache in 1891. The group portrait includes the leaders of the French Egyptology Society, which was headquartered in Cairo at the time. These include archaeologist Georges Émile Jules Daressy (fifth from the left), physician Dr. Guizot (who has begun the unwrapping), and Egyptologist Gaston Maspero (standing in the middle at the far end of the table). A piece of the mummy's shroud and four enamel figurines recovered from her tomb remain sealed under glass in the lower edge of the frame (*Peter Nahum at the Leicester Galleries*).

medicine (Ikram and Dodson 1998 in Scott 2009). Aside from their pulverization by apothecaries, mummies were in high demand as substitutes for scarce cadavers for medical dissection. The legal supply of fresh bodies from the gallows was not enough to satisfy the demand by the burgeoning medical schools in the U.K. and Europe, so an alternative to patronizing the bodysnatchers was the surgical examination of ancient Egyptian bodies. One such event, witnessed by Dr. William Hunter, took place in 1763 in the home of Dr. John Hadley, who conceded that little was learnt due to the poor condition of the mummy, covered as it was in solidified embalming resins (Scott 2009).

Though with today's technology, mummies can be unwrapped by means of non-invasive techniques, museums in the past also resorted to unrollings with varied success to examine their mummies. When Baron Dominique Vivant Denon became the first director of the Louvre, he no doubt intended to research and document the mummies he brought back from his turn-of-the-nineteenth-century trip to Egypt, but they had by then acquired such a foul stench that King Charles X ordered them to be reburied on the grounds of the museum (Sepiel 1996 in Scott 2009). But in 1792, Dr. Johann Friedrich Blumenbach successfully unrolled the first ancient Egyptian mummy accessioned by the British Museum. Two mummies acquired by collector Giuseppe Passalacqua, who became curator of the Berlin Museum's Egyptian Collection, were unrolled in Paris in 1827: one at the Sorbonne and the other — attended by the ambassadors of Prussia, Bavaria, and Tuscany — at the Louvre.

The *New York Times* reported on the unrolling of a mummy by renowned English Egyptologist E.A. Wallis Budge. Budge had been requested to do the honors when curators decided to unwrap the mummy, which had lain in the University museum without provenance for fifty years. A large group of learned men assembled in the botanical theater at University College, London, in December 1889. Budge made some prefatory remarks, then began to unwind yards of thick, yellowish linen that varied in width from four to twelve inches. A slightly disagreeable aromatic odor became more pungent as the unrolling progressed. The linen bands closest to the body were covered with inscriptions that were obscured with bituminous stains. The exposed body was almost black and the skin was hard and shiny. "The features when disclosed stood out very clearly, and were those of a rather handsome person, but the sex could not be determined," reads the account. The arms were stretched out lengthwise on the abdomen and the internal organs had been placed beneath the knees. Artificial eyes had been inserted and the ears had been plugged. Budge estimated the mummy's time period to be the Nineteenth Dynasty, based on the legible inscriptions and the quality of the linen. The mummy was measured at five feet three inches and the account concludes that it would undergo further scientific investigation.

4. Anatomists as Superlatives and Showmen (Thomas Pettigrew)

Several professional demonstrations for the edification and entertainment of the public were performed in the eighteenth and nineteenth centuries, but the trend had truly gathered pace following the supply of mummies which arrived with the return of Napoleon's troops from Egypt in 1801 and the interest garnered by the subsequent "Egyptomania" that swept across England. The mummified remains of an Egyptian female named Irtyersenu had been unwrapped over several weeks in 1821 by Augustus Bozzi Granville, who determined that the woman had died at fifty to fifty-five years of age of ovarian cancer (recently refuted), had given birth, and was overweight. Granville published the results and preserved the viscera, still on display at the British Museum. In 1823, the mummy of a young boy identified as Petamenophis was unwrapped by Frédéric Cailliaud. In 1830, a Twenty-Sixth Dynasty female mummy from Thebes named Irtyru was autopsied by three surgeons on behalf of the Literary and Philosophical Society of Newcastle Upon Tyne, to which it had been donated eight years earlier. The unrolling took place in a lecture theater before "professional gentlemen," and was reported in the local newspapers (Scott 2009). A mummy identified as Takabuti was unwrapped, examined by phrenologists, and reported on by the Belfast Natural History Society in 1835. Dissections open to the general public were conducted by Blumenbach, Giovanni Belzoni, Giovanni Athanasi, and others, and generated significant income for surgeons and professional societies.

Still, members of the audience who had acquired mummies of their own during holidays to Egypt tried their own hand at unwrapping them, conducting soirees at their homes that valued the entertainment value of the private event over the science that the professionals were now seriously pursuing (Dunand and Lichtenberg 2006 in Scott 2009). Doctors and aristocrats were vying for mummies to unwrap for different reasons and the social event did not necessitate documentation. The scientific unrolling, on the other hand, led to the publication of descriptions in journals, proceedings, newspapers, and books; the preservation of specimens; and the attempt at continued conservation of the corpse itself, often by the application of varnish. Although this didn't always leave the remains in condition for reexamination — and countless ancient mummies in both private and professional hands have been lost to history and to science — it did allow Sir Grafton Elliot Smith to x-ray the royal mummy of Tuthmosis IV after it had been unwrapped in a public autopsy by French Egyptologist Gaston Maspero (1846–1916) in 1903. Conversely, the 375 meters of linen shrouding the mummy of Wah (D.C. 2000 B.C.), an estate manager whose sarcophagus was found in 1920, were unwound by his curators at the Metropolitan Museum of Art seventeen years later when x-rays revealed a scarab necklace within.

The man whose name is most associated with social unrolling events is London surgeon Thomas Joseph Pettigrew (1791–1865) — so much so that he became known as "Mummy" Pettigrew. His antiquarian interests overtook his medical pursuits, and he unwrapped dozens of mummies during his lifetime. Unlike many other unrollers, he made careful observations during the process that added to the scholarly study of mummies. Pettigrew's first opportunity to examine mummies came at the request of Italian explorer Giovanni Battista Belzoni. He soon purchased a mummy from a private collection which he unwrapped on his own and at leisure in his home, although he didn't learn much from it because it was in poor condition. Pettigrew then embarked on a series of ceremonious unrollings with audiences present. In April 1833, in the well-attended lecture-theater of Charing Cross Hospital, he unrolled two mummies that he and a friend had purchased at an auction at Sotheby's for a total of less than sixty pounds. A second friend offered a third mummy from the same lot for unwrapping in June of that year. When in July 1833 he assisted an amateur friend unroll a mummy from his collection, this event in the lecture hall at the Royal Institution was documented in a published account, complete with colored plates.

By this time, Pettigrew was working on his own book — the important *History of Egyptian Mummies*— and he was eager to examine the companion mummy, which had gone to the Royal College of Surgeons. "It would be very satisfactory to have the mummy unrolled and this may be done without any injury whatever to the case," he wrote that December. "I should be happy to undertake this task or to assist any one in the performance...." His request was granted, and in mid–January 1834, a ticketed unrolling was conducted before a sold-out crowd of spectators including the trustees of the Hunterian Collection and the British Museum. The mummy was unwrapped "as carefully as circumstances and time permitted." Exposure of part of the face revealed artificial eyes. Particular attention was paid to the linens, some of which showed by their torn edges to have come from larger pieces of cloth. A small scarab was found on the breast and a small clay mummy case was discovered behind the scrotum. Prior to this event — and to add to the research for his book — Pettigrew had witnessed the unrolling of a specimen at the Mechanics' Institution.

After his book's publication, Pettigrew was even more frequently invited to lecture. Dr. John Lee, who had a private museum at Hartwell House, released a mummy for unrolling in May 1836. This event took place over three hours at the Royal Institution. A packed crowd watched as Pettigrew unwrapped the mummy, observing that the linens must have been put on in a damp state and dried by exposing the body to heat. He exposed the incision in the flank through which the viscera had been removed. He demonstrated that the arms had been swathed separately and that some portions of the body had been gilded. And he revealed that the head was bald, indicating that the man was a priest, but that a beard was clearly evident.

In March 1837, Pettigrew delivered to participants — who were willing to pay twice as much for a front-row seat — a six-lecture course in Egyptian antiquities that culminated in a mummy unrolling. A syllabus was issued for the course, which took place in Exeter Hall, Strand. It was reported that a Graeco-Egyptian mummy was provided by Mr. Jones of the Admiralty. The bowels had been extracted through an incision in the left flank, and the brains through the nostrils, as indicated by the broken nose. The arms were crossed over the breast and the mummy wore a thin golden scarab. The eyes, the knees, and the bridge of the nose were topped with gold ornaments. There were rings on the fingers, and the nails of the fingers and toes were gilt. Even though there was not sufficient time to completely unwrap the body, Pettigrew was loudly applauded. At the conclusion, he promoted his *next* unrolling- in April, again in Exeter Hall — which drew another large crowd. The mummy exposed at that event was determined, from the inscriptions, to be an eminent priest. Pieces of linen covered with figures and hieroglyphs had been placed lengthwise down the front of the body, the arms had been crossed over the breast, and the legs had been separately wrapped. The man wore a gilded miter and had gilded nails. Many stone amulets were found about the neck. The mummy itself was encased in a hard layer which "resisted hammers, knives, and chisels," and so was only partially removed. Pettigrew promised the audience of five hundred that the task would be undertaken elsewhere and submitted to public view.

With his fame now at its height, Pettigrew repeated his six-lecture course on the island of Jersey in August 1837. To conclude the course, he unrolled the "Jersey Mummy," which had been presented to the Jersey Museum after the man who purchased it in Egypt, John Gossett, had died on his way home. The Jersey Mummy had been adorned with a garland of lotus flowers. As the linens were unrolled, "the room became filled with a strong but not very disagreeable odour." An inner layer saturated with resin had to be picked apart, but revealed wrappings with a colored border which, when lifted, hid a fine scarab ornament. The mummy was then lifted and carried around the audience so everyone could have a good look, which each stood to do. When the unrolling commenced, Pettigrew announced a further surprise: the discovery of a novel ornament consisting of a scarab atop a metal plate in the form of a hawk with expanded wings and ankhs in his talons. The ornament was handed around the audience, who registered their admiration with applause. The excited audience next applauded the freeing of the black and shriveled left foot from its wrappings.... Pettigrew carried out further examinations of the Jersey Mummy after the lecture and his results were reported in the press. His unusual findings included the replacement of the cleaned and purified organs within the body cavity and the substitution of the brain with sand through an incision in the throat rather than through the nose.

Pettigrew presented a paper on the Jersey Mummy to the Society of Antiquaries in November 1837, but then devoted several years to his professional practice and to writing a biography. It wasn't until January 1840 that he returned to unrolling — this time of the daughter of a priest at the Islington Literary and Scientific Institute. The event was reported in the newspaper, but not with the same vigor as earlier accounts: "The only ornaments found on the antiquated dame were a few common beads and a ring. That she was old before she died the state of the teeth gave proof. The Mummy had been brought from Thebes, and presents the characteristics usually observed in the embalming of that locality." The report — if not the event itself — seems rather tedious.

A more exciting demonstration was made in 1843 at the first annual congress of the British Archaeological Association that Pettigrew had been instrumental in founding. The unrolling was held at the Canterbury Theatre, where the orchestra pit had been boarded over and the stage outfitted with appropriate and imposing decorations. All boxes were filled and Pettigrew began with an hour-long lecture. He then began the unrolling of a mummy whose name had been translated as "Har son of Unefer" and which Pettigrew had purchased in London. He and his son T.J. removed the resinous linens by cutting them away with knives. The work took an hour before revealing the form of the body and a "complacent smile" on the face. Bits of wrapping, although they had a peculiar and disagreeable smell, were circulated among the audience members, who also breathed in the dust that had been created. Pettigrew sawed off the back of the skull to find it had been filled with pitch. At the end of the three-hour performance, "the mummy, which proved to be that of a young man, was raised to its feet, and presented to the company, and was received with enthusiastic applause." Presumably, members of the satisfied audience were allowed to take away the pieces of linen as souvenirs.

The dramatic event at Canterbury was followed up in 1848 in the Shire Hall at the Worcester Congress. Pettigrew was provided with a mummy to unroll by Joseph Arden. He was assisted by his son during the three-hour demonstration, which began with another hour-long lecture. In May 1851, Pettigrew performed his last public unrolling: that of a specimen belonging to the United Service Institution, with printed announcements issued to members of the organization. It was noted that the viscera, accompanied by wax figures of their guardian deities, had been wrapped and placed between the legs. "Mummy" Pettigrew's legacy had been secured: He was parodied in *Punch* and became the subject of verse:

> E'en on that sink of all iniquity, the Stage,
> The sacrilegious monsters dared engage
>   On Friday evening to strip a corse —
>   A Mummy called they it — and what was worse,

> Sawed through the head — as it had been a cheese;
> (Praise be where due, the powder made them sneeze)
> Then placed upon its feet the insulted dead,
> Gave three wild yells, called cheers — and went to bed.

This was in reference to the Canterbury event, at which the satisfied crowd did not leave the auditorium until the late hour of 11 P.M.

While the trend got off to a later start, mummy unrollings were conducted in America, but usually before a smaller scholarly crowd. The first public unwrapping was done in front of an audience of faculty and "respectable citizens" in Castle Garden in New York City, on December 14, 1824. Bandages were cut through the back and separated from the female mummy, which exposed her body to view (Wolfe 2009). Pains were taken to ensure there was no fakery. When Philadelphia merchant John L. Hodge imported a mummy in June 1825 and unrolled it that year, the examination included a medical inspection to make sure the mummy was authentic. Two mummies purchased by Rubens Peale were unwrapped on March 3, 1826, in a lecture room of his museum and were inspected by two doctors before being placed on display. Peale's rival, John Scudder of the American Museum, offered fifty tickets to an unrolling in January 1832, displaying the mummy before and after the event. And an audience of medical students, scientific gentlemen, and theologians observed a mummy unrolling by Dr. J.H. Miller in December 1838 at the Medical College of Baltimore (Wolfe 2009).

Rather than just private after-dinner parlor amusements, most of the mummy unrollings in the U.S. were conducted under the auspices of institutions of learning, although it was acknowledged that more than just intellectual curiosity drew some audience members. A New Orleans newspaper wrote, "Apart from the mere curiosity to witness the mere operation of unrolling a mummy, which motives will doubtless attract many spectators, the novel and instructive explanations that will accompany it will be an attraction equally powerful and of useful results." The subject of the report was an 1851 unrolling at the University of Louisiana performed by three members of the medical faculty, after which the findings were written up and the mummy placed in the school's medical museum. In December of 1864, tickets to an unrolling at the New York Historical Society were sold for fifty cents each and the mummy was unwrapped by a professor as part of a series of lectures on ancient Egypt. Another mummy was unwrapped by a demonstrator of anatomy at Columbia University, and yet another was revealed before an audience of 150 at Cornell (Wolfe 2009).

While Britain's "Mummy" Pettigrew gained his fame by unwrapping mummies, popular American Egyptologist George Robins Gliddon (1809–1857) *lost* his reputation during a highly publicized mummy unrolling. He had begun lecturing on Egyptian art and artifacts in the U.S. in the 1840s, after returning from his post as vice-consul in Cairo. He always appeared dressed in black and dramatized his lectures with 800-foot revolving backdrops of exotic scenes from the Nile Valley. He packed the lecture halls and impressed his audiences with scientific-sounding oratory. To satisfy public curiosity about mummies, Gliddon ordered a dozen from an Egyptian dealer who obtained them by looting the tombs around modern Luxor. Most were lost in a Nile flood, but the two that were supplied dated to 900 B.C. and were said to have originated in ancient Thebes. Gliddon translated their sarcophagi to indicate they were a pair of Egyptian priestesses and announced the unwrapping of "Got Thothi Aunk" and "Nefer Atethu" as an unprecedented event. When the papers misinterpreted "priestess" as "princess," he chose not to correct them. Through advance publicity, he secured 250 subscriptions (which allowed the bearer to four tickets each) at five dollars each. He formed a committee of seventeen medical and scientific men to supervise the process.

In Boston in 1850, before a capacity crowd of 2,000 physicians and intellectuals — including Henry Wadsworth Longfellow, Oliver Wendell Holmes, and Louis Agassiz — Gliddon proceeded with his presentation. The unwrapping began during the first lecture, but the surprise did not occur until the third. "As he unrolled the linen and pulled off the last sheet, it was very apparent that the mummy was a man.... Everybody laughed at Gliddon and his fame collapsed. It was a fiasco," explains Guido Lombardi, an anthropology student who documented the story as part of his master's thesis. Though not accused of deliberate deception, Gliddon was ridiculed in local and national newspapers. He left town for Philadelphia and sold subscriptions to another series of lectures featuring the unrolling of two mummies, the second of which had been so heavily embalmed that the wrappings had to be breached at a later well-attended event. Gliddon used the mummies from his infamous Boston lecture series — a male and a female, as it turned out — to demonstrate racially misguided theories of craniology before donating them in 1851 and 1852 to Tulane University (at the time called the University of Louisiana), where they have resided ever since. And it was in New Orleans in 1852 that Gliddon offered to unwrap his last mummy.

Unrollings typically took a couple of hours, such as the 1887 unwrapping of a mummy at the New Brunswick Theological Seminary by a professor, a doctor, and seminary librarian. But occasionally the embalming resins thwarted the demonstrations — or at least made them rather unpleasant. In September 1895, Dr. Goucher had to abort attempts to unwrap a mummy at Women's College in Baltimore because the bundle had completely solidified *and he had to catch his train home* (Wolfe 2009). Dr. J.G. Lansing had varying degrees of success unrolling one of two mummies that had been imported in 1888. With professors and clergy present at the now-defunct George West Museum, a choir sang, the bishop gave a prayer and address, and Dr. Lansing delivered a short lecture about embalming. Then he and some associates took the cover off the box, removed all but the innermost wrappings which adhered to the mummy, and laid the mummy on a table. They had to yank on the remaining wrappings and go at them with a carving knife. As they pared away, small boys ran off with bits and women turned away at the smell. The embalming was found to have been badly done, but nevertheless they managed to uncover the head to reveal a full set of teeth and unwrap the female mummy to the waist so photographs could be made. The mummy's feet had broken off during transport and hung by the wrappings — until one of them fell to the platform (Wolfe 2009). Another unrolling with religious trappings was less noteworthy, but distinct because it is one of the few recorded instances of an American unwrapping party. In Lincoln, Nebraska, in 1892, twenty-one new members of the Grace Lutheran Church were treated to an exhibit of a number of mummies that had been imported at great expense for the party by Mr. and Mrs. C.J. Ernst (Wolfe 2009).

Mummy unwrapping continued into the twentieth century in the U.K. and abroad. Sir Grafton Elliot Smith's career took a big leap forward when he was commissioned by the Egyptian government in 1907 to investigate antiquities endangered by the Aswan Dam project. Among the 30,000 mummy examinations he was said to have performed were the autopsies of 2,000 threatened mummies (Cockburn 1980 in Scott 2009). These were hurried, apparently private, and poorly recorded. Meanwhile, a mummy autopsy of two Twelfth-Dynasty brothers had been undertaken in 1908 by a collaboration of scientists at the Manchester Museum, and their remains — skeletonized for the most part — are on display in the museum's galleries. The next unwrapping of an ancient Egyptian mummy in England did not occur until 1975, again at the Manchester Museum. Billed as "the most extensive examination of its kind to have been carried out in Britain," the event was filmed by the BBC for a television docu-

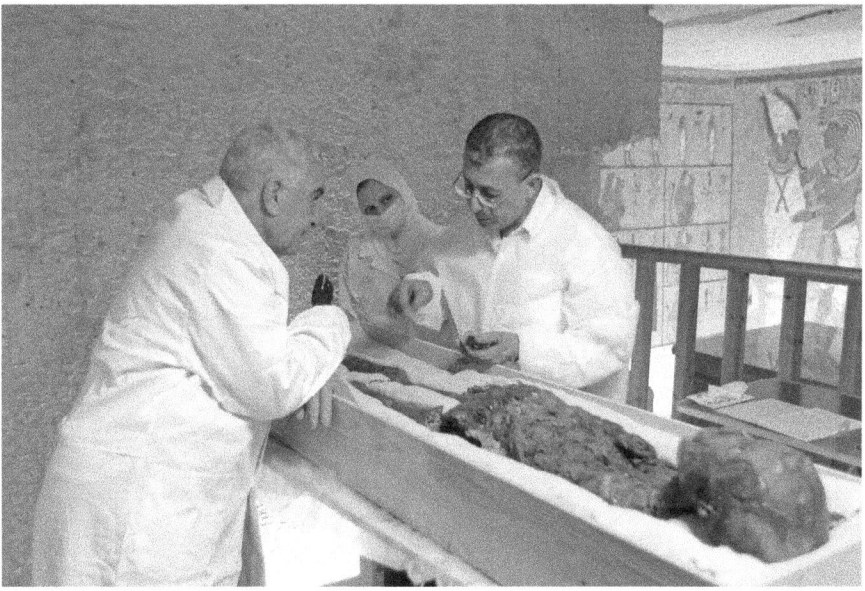

Dr. Zahi Hawass, Secretary General of the Supreme Council of Antiquities in Cairo, and Dr. Yehia Zakaria Gad of the Department of Medical Molecular Genetics at Cairo's National Research Center examine and remove DNA samples from the mummy of Egyptian pharaoh Tutankhamun in his tomb in Luxor in 2007. Results of the genetic testing, revealed in 2010, confirmed family relationships and elucidated the pharaoh's medical history. King Tut's mummy had been unwrapped by Howard Carter's team after the discovery of the tomb in 1922 (*Barry Iverson Photography*).

mentary and by Manchester University for two teaching films. The following year, the mummy of Pharaoh Ramesses II, which had been unwrapped by Maspero in Egypt in the late 1800s, underwent comprehensive study, restoration, and conservation by a team of twenty researchers who completed a complete examination and a battery of tests and analyses.

With interest generated by the Manchester autopsy and the Paris conservation work, the Bristol Museum — which had not unwrapped a mummy since 1830 — undertook in 1981 the reexamination and conservation of the preserved remains of Horemkenesi, which had been discovered in Deir el Bahri in 1904–05. As with the Paris examination, the results were published in a book. After that, in 1985, the Guimet Museum of Natural History in Lyons, France, unwrapped and studied an ancient mummy using modern medical equipment (El Mahdy 1989 in Scott 2009). These were among the last physical mummy unwrapping in the U.K. and Europe. With the advances in imaging, the destructive unrollings of yesterday have been made obsolete. But the unwrapping of mummies in earlier centuries was questioned then and now. With the budding interest in ethnology, there was a misguided attempt by craniologist Samuel George Morton and others to demonstrate that the black race did not descend from the "magnificent culture" of the ancient Egyptians (Wolfe 2009). That unwrappings were well-attended by a lay and learned audience and were widely reported in newspapers was evidence that they garnered both a scientific and a prurient interest. But comments in those same newspapers about the unrollings indicate that at least some people were disturbed that the remains of a human being had been treated so cavalierly and irreverently. Some wondered what would become of the soul with the body so far-removed from Egypt, and some saw the public demonstrations as an affront to any corpse (Wolfe 2009).

P.T. Barnum (1810–1891) and His Hoax

Joice Heth was billed by American showman P.T. Barnum as "the greatest national and natural curiosity in the world." She was said to have been born in 1674, to have nursed future president George Washington while she was a slave, and to be on tour in 1835 at the age of 161. Even though she was blind, toothless, nearly paralyzed, and toured with Barnum for only seven months, Heth springboarded his career after he purchased her for $1,000 from her former promoter R.W. Lindsay. He was eager to become the proprietor of this novel exhibition, says Barnum in his autobiography, and writes, "At the outset of my career I saw that everything depended upon getting the people to think, and talk, and become curious and excited over and about the 'rare spectacle.' Accordingly, posters, transparencies, advertisements, and newspaper paragraphs — all calculated to extort attention — were employed, regardless of expense" (Barnum 1888). Heth's act — which consisted of telling stories about "little George," singing hymns, and entertaining questions from the audience — raked in a handsome profit for the showman. She performed for as long as twelve hours a day, six days a week, in everything from museums and concert halls to taverns and railway houses across the northeastern United States.

Her twelve-page show history (*The Life of Joice Heth* 1835), which circulated at the time for a price of six cents, fictionalized Heth's history, stating that she had been imported to America from Madagascar at the age of fifteen. She managed both the kitchen and the nursery of the Washington home, and the family entrusted her and treated her more like a hired servant than a slave. According to the pamphlet, not only was Heth the first person to swaddle baby George, she had given birth to fifteen children of her own. When she reached the age of fifty-four, she was sold to the owner of her husband Peter so that the couple could live out their years together with a lighter workload. After her husband and her owner died, she was passed down to various heirs and was for lengths of time neglected as she became more infirm. Her hearing, though, was said to be fine, and she was bright, animated, and pious. She had never taken medicine, and smoked tobacco out of a pipe. The show history proclaims that she was much happier in her present situation and was fed adequately and provided with a nurse to look after her. The newspaper accounts quoted in the document describe her as a "living mummy" with fingers "like the talons of a bird of prey." Lastly, the show history explains that she is working to buy the freedom of the only of her descendants she has not outlived: five great-grandchildren enslaved in Kentucky.

Doubts were raised repeatedly in the press about the authenticity of Heth's age and even her person (it was claimed that she was an automaton). With much of the controversy stirred up by Barnum himself to reignite flagging interest, the showman promised a postmortem examination. After Heth died of natural causes on February 19, 1836, Barnum engaged the services of surgeon David L. Rogers to perform an autopsy "in the presence of some medical students," as he describes (Barnum 1888). In fact, the showman sold 1,500 tickets at fifty cents apiece to members of the public willing to pay for the privilege of witnessing Heth's dissection in New York's City. Although Barnum (1888) later stated that doctors disagreed about the meaning of the body's lack of ossification, Dr. Rogers declared the age claim a fraud, pronouncing that she was probably no older than eighty. At this, Barnum insisted that there had been a case of mistaken identity and that Heth was still alive. Later he admitted the hoax.

Gunther von Hagens (1945–) and His Spectacles

Gunther von Hagens, the anatomist most likely to be remembered from our age, prides himself on his homage to the past. When he performed a controversial public dissection in 2002, he wore a black fedora echoing the hat worn by Dr. Nicolaes Tulp in Rembrandt's famous seventeenth-century painting, a reproduction of which hung overhead. Tulp, possibly to be seen as his successor, patterned himself after Vesalius, who is shown dissecting a forearm and hand in the frontispiece of history's most famous medical textbook. With his static full-body preparations, von Hagens most closely parallels eighteenth-century French anatomist Honoré Fragonard. They have both succeeded in preserving entire selectively-dissected cadavers, and they have both been criticized: "No preparation, even executed with the greatest care, holds to me any value if it does not demonstrate a new fact or the resolution of a debated issue. All their preparations ... satisfy only the gaze; few among them serve to demonstrate any new truths, to refute old errors; the refinements throughout are not instructive and demonstrate only the handiwork of their creator" (Degueurce 2011). This was not the remark of one of the millions of people to visit von Hagens' BodyWorlds exhibits since 1994 — although it easily could be. It was said of Fragonard's cabinet by German physician Georg Ludwig Rumpelt in 1779.

The way von Hagens preserves his cadavers is through an innovative process he developed and patented in the 1990s and calls "plastination." He forcibly replaces the fluid and fats in the bodies with a reactive polymer which makes them dry, odorless, durable, and completely stable. They are selectively dissected, arranged in the desired position, and gas-cured so that they will harden and can stand unsupported. The resulting sculptural corpses do and don't follow precedent. The plastination method results in vibrant coloration, which the earlier anatomists were only able to achieve in illustrations or with models. The famous "auto-icon" of philosopher Jeremy Bentham, to which the plastinates have been compared (Pierson 2009), is hardly as colorful or lifelike. Plastinating cadavers eliminates the need to mediate between viewer and body, even with a display case. Patrons of the exhibits are asked not to touch the specimens, but are otherwise free to examine them as closely as they wish, a freedom earlier visitors to anatomical museums did not have.

In his exhibition catalog, von Hagens (Anatomy 2004) explains that anatomist Andreas Vesalius "pulled the dead out of their graves and put them back in society" by assembling human bones into upright structures he called skeletons, a revolutionary idea at the time which we now take for granted. In the *New York Times*, Mary Ore (2002) suggests that by solidifying soft tissue and incorporating muscle tissue, fat, and organs, von Hagens "has taken the skeleton to its natural conclusion." Portraying the dead human body as alive through his novel method of plastination follows an old anatomical tradition. While cadavers undergo reductive dissection that leaves them looking undoubtedly dead, representations of cadavers (in drawings, for instance) are depicted as living beings, often participating in their own dissection (Jones 2002). Deanna Petheridge (Petheridge and Jordanova 1997) calls it one of the most persistent visual conventions in anatomical art.

With the advent of plastination, a new level of dynamism of the dead has been achieved. At von Hagens' whim, his cadavers are poised swimming in mid-stroke, kicking a soccer ball, running, dancing, and a number of other activities. With plastination an unsurpassed means of presenting the most "alive" dead body possible, von Hagens consciously recreates the anatomical art of earlier centuries as part of that tradition and to show what the early anatomists showed in an improved way. The plastinated man holding his skin is — minus the knife — a direct remediation of a sixteenth-century Juan de Valverde drawing showing a man as if he has just survived skinning himself. A reclining man whose muscles are highlighted is the plastinated incarnation of the classic sculptural pose of the "flayed man," who has been translated to paper, plaster, bronze — and now posterity. Von Hagens also draws heavily on the wax figures prepared in Italy in the eighteenth and nineteenth centuries. Figures like the reclining pregnant woman owe their creation and reception in part to the way the famous Venus models exposed their organs, including their wombs.

With some of his preserved cadavers, von Hagens has mimicked the anatomical art of earlier centuries. He replicates Honoré Fragonard's nineteenth-century "myologies," but even more impressively models his "Man on Horseback" after the horse and rider Fragonard embalmed. Von Hagens deliberately reproduces the preparations of the past, but sometimes his anatomical exercises *unintentionally* echo history. His satisfaction at plastinating a reclining woman in the eighth month of pregnancy, and his attention to surface details like female nipples, mirror the delight experienced by centuries of earlier anatomists at the prospect of dissecting a rare female cadaver. Stephen Johnson (2009) states that BodyWorlds preserves — though not overtly — the features that characterized the Victorian anatomical museum, including the display of authentic specimens, physical aberrations, and sexuality. The lifelike attitudes of the plastinates leave them vulnerable to criticisms that they appeal (purposely or not) to a prurient gaze. The reclining pregnant plastinate, although a deliberate remediation of the classic wax "Venus" figure, is criticized (as the original was) for her sexually seductive pose. In fact, most of the full-body plastinates are male, but the exposure of the genitals of both genders is excused by establishing them as objects under study. In other words, voyeurism is allowed if it is educational.

Where objectivity defines traditional anatomical exhibits, the posthumous personalities of the plastinates draws the crowds. Von Hagens' stated aim is to democratize anatomy — to allow laypeople direct access to the authentic interior of the human body. He does not intend plastinates to be perceived objectively, like most museum specimens, but to elicit an emotional response. Plastination solves the problems that have plagued anatomists for centuries — plastinates are real bodies, but do not decay or discolor. "From the time of Vesalius to the days of von Hagens, we see anatomists struggling to combine a preference for authentic bodies with the educational advantages of body models" (van Dijck 2001). Plastination achieves that, to an almost overwhelming degree. Jose van Dijck (2001) reasons, "The plastinated cadaver is thus as much an organic artifact as it is the result of technological tooling." The terminology chosen to describe plastinated bodies captures their authenticity, while at the same time assimilating their role as anatomical models, which are more often not real. Plastinates have been referred to as "reconfigurations" rather than imitations. They are said to be dissected, preserved, and "recomposed." Van Dijck (2001) calls those whose poses mimic earlier anatomical illustrations "reanimations of representations." Von Hagens explains that the root of his word "plastination" is from the Greek plassein, meaning to mold or form (2004). The consensus is that plastinates are modified bodies, but bodies nonetheless.

But to assuage the layperson's "visceral reaction" to being in a room with so many bodies, von Hagens exercises tight control of the experience. He stages his shows in science museums, allying his dissections with medicine to gain legitimacy and justifying the provocative poses of his plastinates. He provides the public with a spectacle, but makes his figures conform to established principles of aesthetics (no missing teeth or limbs, for instance), so that they shock, but not too much. By abandoning clinical detachment, von Hagens does away with objectivity, and has therefore been accused of stepping out of the bounds of science. His plastinates are — like cadavers — anonymous, but in clinical practice bodies do not have aesthetic qualities and von Hagens' plastinates do. They are no longer objective specimens and that changes the way they are looked at: "The greater the artistic license in the poses, the less clinical the exhibits become, and the less legitimate they become, for some visitors," says Tony Walter (2004a).

Von Hagens' preparations often draw more attention to plastination itself than to the organs and systems they are used to demonstrate, a reaction upon which he capitalizes. One of the ways the anatomist deflects criticism that he is using the human body to create art is by sharing the secrets of his preservative method, which many of his predecessors were reluctant to do. He even claims that it offers the body donors life after death, promising, "Plastination is thus able to satisfy the desire for immortality, which until now has been monopolized by the Church, in a way that is commensurate with our times" (2004b). Even so, these are incorruptible anatomical specimens (Brock 2004), not memorialized lives, by virtue of their anonymity. And yet they do have individual presence, with each distinct body intended to represent a universal anatomy. The anatomist has stripped them of their skin and thereby their identity, but has repersonalized them by adding surface details like eyes and by posing them with props. Tony Walter (2004b) points this out:

> So, there is a contradiction: the exhibition shows the human body with clinical, impersonal, scientific detachment, yet at the same time breaks with twentieth-century anatomy not only in showing human remains to the public but in giving them spectacularly individual and playful identities.

Anonymity downplays what the unique poses bring up, and we cannot see plastinates as either individuals or universals, because they are both.

Von Hagens often has to counter accusations that he is a sculptor of human clay. In a video projection at the BodyWorlds exhibition in Mannheim, he was shown carving away body fat and chiseling a body into shape, much like a sculptor (van Dijck 2005). The scientific specimens he prepares express his personality, which is usually characteristic of art, and he consistently adopts the identity of an artist (van Dijck 2001). In fact, although he eschews being called an artist, he acknowledges his creative role and laments (von Hagens, 2004a) that dissection has lost its creative components. His critics argue that his talents are far from uplifting in today's world:

> Stripping away the layers of skin and flesh and bone "beneath the surface" of our bodies does not bring us any closer to the essence of our humanity, which is to be found in a quite different place: in that most

distinctive of human creations, our civilization. The emergence of the mutilated body as a public spectacle reflects the degradation of contemporary humanity at a time when there is widespread disillusionment with the state of our society and its prospects for the future [Fitzpatrick 2002].

The BodyWorlds exhibitions are accused of appealing to morbid curiosity. Von Hagens is well aware of the emotional reactions of the viewers, acknowledges morbid curiosity, and admits that some of the specimens are difficult to look at (Jeffries 2002). This is partly explained by Ludmilla Jordanova, who points out that figures which are half skeleton and half flesh are — because they evoke the passage from life to death — even more forceful than the iconic skeletal memento mori (Petheridge and Jordanova 1997). So although the anatomist focuses on the demonstrated living capabilities of the body, using dynamism as a distancing device, the presence of death in such quantity is moving, prompting art critic Lucas Carpenter (2001) to refer to the exhibit's collective memento mori effect. The didactic intent of the exhibit is obscured by this shock value and by its positioning within today's entertainment industry. Attempts to locate BodyWorlds strictly within the arena of education, art, or amusement is futile. As José van Dijk (2001) notes: "From the history of anatomy we have learned that the anatomical practices, objects, and representations have always been an intricate mixture of science and art, and a hybrid of medical instruction and popular entertainment." As with most gallery experiences, establishing a relationship with the plastinates in the BodyWorlds exhibition takes only a few minutes. Their friendly poses invite curiosity and the craft in their presentation leaves little room for horror or disgust.

The assembled troupe of full-body preparations have not been hidden away in the anatomist's "cabinet," but taken on tour. Each of his BodyWorlds exhibits includes roughly two dozen plastinates, which alternate in the viewer's mind as cadavers and as sculptures. The results of his anatomically informed imagination are unique, which usually characterizes an original work of art. Although von Hagens allies himself with the scientific community and promotes the plastinates as educational three-dimensional illustrations, their sculptural quality continues to overshadow their instructional value. One specimen shows the black lungs of a smoker, while the next mimics the human figure in a painting by Salvador Dali. Plastination allows what until now has been a feature of two-dimensional drawings: combining in one view what could only be seen in several (Kemp and Wallace 2000). One particularly striking way von Hagens exploits this flexibility is to create more than one figure from a single body. One plastinated specimen, for instance, consists of a muscleman being tapped on his shoulder by his own skeleton. There is no denying that the technique is more proficient and efficient than any that have gone before, especially when one considers that a single classic drawing or model could involve the successive dissection of dozens of bodies to complete.

The portrayal of the show as "something to see" is done largely through the meticulous public relations campaigns of Gunther von Hagens. From the poses he chooses to the photographs he releases to the media, the anatomist himself serves as mediator between anatomic information and the public. Von Hagens decides which plastinates will be seen. His European shows included deformed fetuses, which have been left out of the show as it tours the United States. He will not display plastinated children, although he has body donors as young as six years old. The anatomist successfully navigates the fine lines between art and science, between dignified and exploitive, and his success is measured in the number of tickets he has sold, the amount of newspaper copy he has generated, and the attention he has garnered as the impresario of his anatomical circus:

> Von Hagens would deny that his edifying exhibit is a sideshow, and to a great extent he would be correct. BodyWorlds is much closer to the narrative of the museum, which downplays sensationalism in the service of educating the public. However, in the regulated sensationalism of the displays, in the power of its discourse that attempts to work on the bodies of its "inmates"—whether the bodies themselves or the bodies of those who pay to see them—in the way it extols the individuals even as individual difference is reduced to an accident of anatomy, BodyWorlds can arguably lay claim to the title of Greatest Show on Earth [Ponce 2009].

Von Hagens welcomed the press, good or bad, from the start and is known to be a self-promoter: "...he has not been overly concerned with keeping his own white coat from flying open to reveal a showman's red vest" (Lara 2005).

Von Hagens renews his shows by adding new plastinates to them, and he keeps himself and his plastination method in the public eye by placing his anatomical entities in venues outside his BodyWorlds shows. Von Hagens appeared with some of his full-body specimens on BBC's period reality TV series "Regency House Party" in 2004, and plastinates made a cameo appearances in the 2006 James Bond film "Casino Royale." Most recently, he is working with American performer Lady Gaga to feature plastinates on the set of her world tour. He consistently stirs up public opinion about his work. He has stated ambitions to reporters that include establishing a permanent museum containing thousands of plastinates, dissecting his father upon his death, and filming the death and plastination of a terminally ill patient. He recently raised the bar of public outrage by posing a male and female corpse in the act of having sex, as part of his display of plastinates entitled "Cycle of Life," which opened in Berlin in 2009. The exhibit was been condemned as indecent and offensive, and German politicians called for it to be withdrawn. Social Democrat Fritz Felegentreu was quoted, "Love and death are obvious topics for art but I find it quite disgusting to use them in this way" ("Gunther von Hagens Exhibition Criticised" 2009). His sentiments were echoed by Alice Strover, a Green party representative, who called the installation "over the top" and said it should not be shown. Von Hagens defended the piece, insisting that the body donors consented to the pose and that it is not intended to be sexually stimulating.

To maintain their existence, museums have to draw crowds and it is exhibits like BodyWorlds that do so. As Elaine Heumann Gurian clarifies, "Museum professionals do not want to be in show business, we want to be in academia. And yet, like it or not, exhibitions are in part public entertainment" (Karp and Lavine 1991). Anatomical cadavers are rarely the objects of public concern and plastination makes them so. Plastinates are presented to the public in spectacular fashion and with controversial editorial discourse, both of which beckon visitors. Von Hagens and his collaborators have developed an economically and socially viable stage on which to make at least visual meaning of the body, and this alone makes it a spectacle. Criticisms of the BodyWorlds exhibition often fall back on arguments that it is in bad taste. The shows have been accused of being tacky and vulgar (Fitzpatrick 2002). Von Hagens circumvents authoritarian strictures of good taste by appealing directly to a mass audience. The exhibition purposely rejects the long-standing distinction between the body's beautiful exterior (represented to the public in art) and its ugly interior (restricted from public view). The people filing past the plastinates are not watching out of an interest in engaging with broad philosophical concepts about being human. What they are really attracted by is the spectacle of real bodies displayed inside out (Miah 2004). "Modern medicine has hidden bodies in hospitals and universities, and I give them back," he is quoted as saying (Singh 2003).

But to keep the visitors coming back, the show must change. Presently von Hagens has three touring exhibitions and a staff of 200 preparing plastinates in creative new poses. His eccentricities are tolerated because his plastination method is truly revolutionary. Although German anatomists tried to expel von Hagens from their profession and British officials tried to deny him an official exhibition permit, his technique is well-respected by anatomists. The display of his plastinates has provoked animated discussions and the occasional incidence of civil disobedience (one plastinate was covered with a blanket, another pummeled with a hammer). The show has even benefited by favorable comparisons with several copycat exhibits that have been mounted, including one in which the specimens were poorly preserved.

The characterization of inventor Gunther von Hagens by the press feeds into the publicity he generates around himself and his publicly exhibited dissections. The media contributed to the success of BodyWorlds, but could not resist the temptation to show the exhibits as well as their creator in a demonic light (Bauer 2004). Accusations that the bodies von Hagens uses have been less than freely donated and, in some cases, obtained after judicial executions, echo the days when anatomists procured their raw material from grave and gallows. Von Hagens does not shy away from media portrayal as a ghoul and that is a large part of the success of his exhibit. He has been called Dr. Death, Frankenstein, the modern Mengele, the Galileo of anatomy. He has been referred to as merely a technically proficient taxidermist (Padley 2003) and has been accused of letting art and artifice overshadow instruction. Some say pre-

4. Anatomists as Superlatives and Showmen (Gunther von Hagens)

senting bodies in lifelike poses makes him more sick-minded sculptor than scientist, more entertainer than teacher (Haithman). "It is an honour to cause this controversy," says von Hagens (Jeffries 2002) as he promotes both himself and his technique.

Admittedly, von Hagens is a showman, but so were the dissectors of the past. English surgeon Sir Astley Cooper bragged to a committee of the House of Commons that he could obtain the body of any person for dissection if he so desired. French naturalist Georges Cuvier was delighted to entertain his colleagues with a view of the legendary genitals of the "Hottentot Venus" which the young woman was too modest to expose to them during live examinations. And when asked about his embalmed full-body adult and infant specimens, French anatomist Honoré Fragonard tantalizingly invited, "Come and see." The preserved anatomy that Gunther von Hagens offers to the public, whether they are interested in medicine or just morbidly curious, should be viewed in the context of the unruly public dissections of the seventeenth and eighteenth centuries. His lure of the crowd should be compared to that of P.T. Barnum, who sold tickets to the autopsy of one of his famous performers. And his passing a tray of organs around the audience of his controversial 2002 public autopsy should be weighed against renowned London surgeon Thomas Joseph Pettigrew circulating bits of the wrapping of the ancient Egyptian mummy he had just "unrolled" before a mesmerized audience.

The plastinated bodies in the BodyWorlds exhibitions startle and provoke, and Gunther von Hagens welcomes the reaction. "What's wrong with sensationalism?" he asks (Bohannon et al. 2003). The bodies are posed in unsettling ways, never purely to shock. Although shock they do, as a claimed byproduct of their informational purpose. José van Dijck (2001) writes, "It is striking how von Hagens reinfuses the element of spectacle into the display — stipulating viewers' 'visceral' identification with the dissected bodies." Some believe that the means is effective, others feel that the message is being overwhelmed by the means. Either way, von Hagens is on a trajectory in which exhibits become ever more exotic as technical possibilities expand and his team dreams up more spectacular poses (Walter 2004a). And the exhibits draw crowds, whether they are there to gawk, to learn, or to consider a new way to spend eternity.

Announcing to the German press shortly before his sixty-sixth birthday in January 2011 that he has been battling Parkinson's disease. von Hagens plans to add to his accomplishments. Anticipating the decline in his ability to manage a large organization, he is scaling down his operations so that he can pursue his scientific goals on an accelerated timeline. In addition to continuing his work on the BodyWorlds exhibitions, he plans to develop a digital anatomical atlas as a contemporary equivalent of Vesalius' *Fabrica,* to file patents for numerous anatomical technologies he has considered for decades, and to document his research and inventions. "I would also like to create a new body of work reconciling human anatomy and art — a continuation of the work of the Renaissance anatomists that I am calling 'aesthetic anatomy,' for exhibitions destined for art museums," he said ("BodyWorlds Creator" 2010). Furthermore, he intends to become one of the anatomical figures in his BodyWorlds exhibits when the degenerative disease eventually results in his death. He intends for his wife and curator of the exhibit Angelina Whalley to plastinate his body. "My plastinated corpse will then stand in a welcoming pose at the entrance of my exhibition. I want to be able to welcome my guests even after I am dead," he explains (Erlanger 2011). If this suggests he is an exhibitionist, that's *exactly* what he is.

In a more historical way of taking the stage, on November 20, 2002, German anatomist Gunther von Hagens conducted what he promoted as the first public autopsy in a century. From 7:00 to 10:00 P.M., some 400 people crowded into a 200-seat auditorium adjacent to the London BodyWorlds exhibition. The attendees had been randomly chosen and the autopsy was a ticketed event, although only a minority had to pay the nineteen-dollar fee. Von Hagens said he regarded his audience as "newcomers" to the science of anatomy, although they were a mix of laypeople and medical students. He was assisted by a German and an English doctor, one of whom recited a brief medical history of the

Opposite: German anatomist Gunther von Hagens sold tickets to the public to observe the dissection of the body of a 72-year-old man, which stirred as much controversy as the display of plastinated corpses in his BodyWorlds exhibits. The event, billed as "Britain's first public autopsy in 172 years," was held in London on November 20, 2002 (*AFP/Getty Images*).

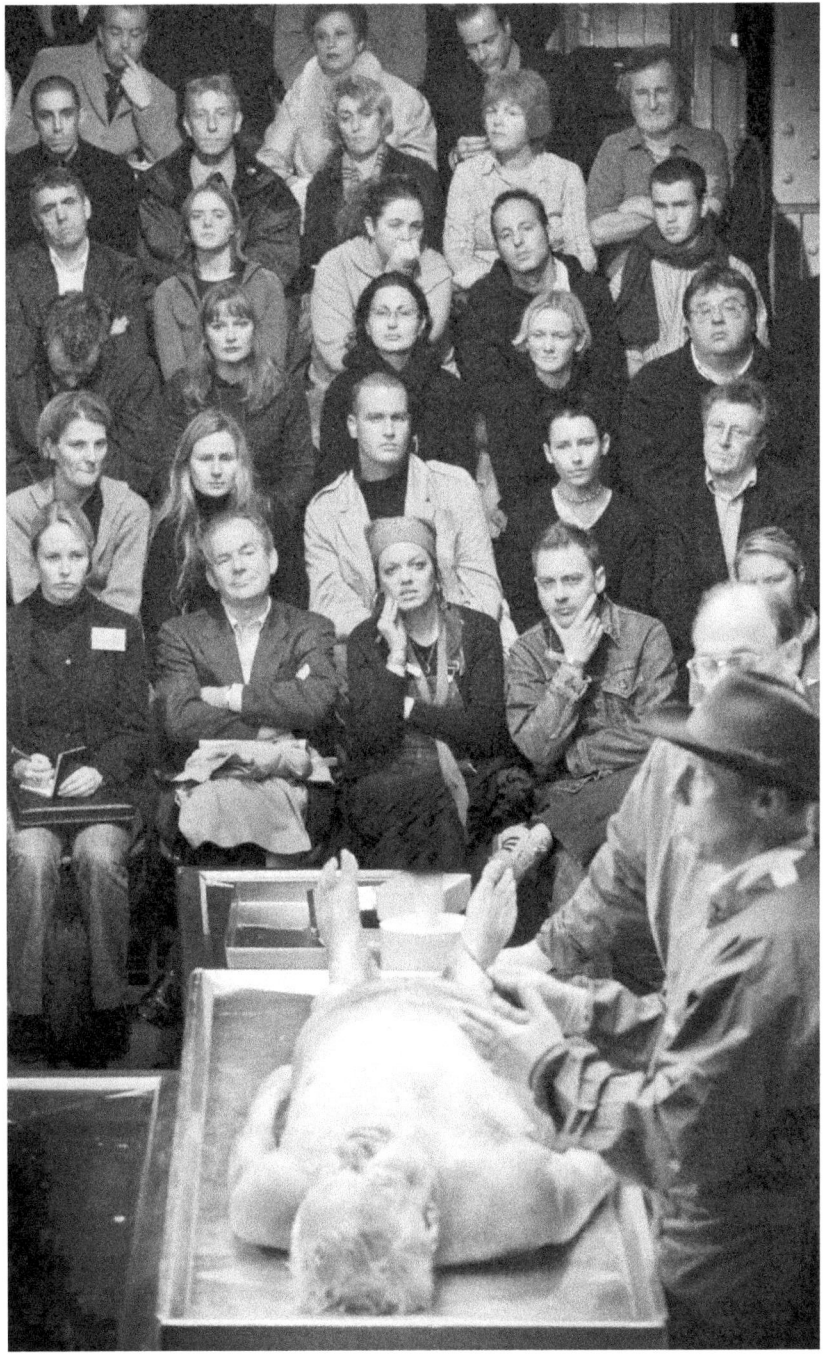

cadaver. The man was a German, seventy-two years of age. He had lost his job as a businessman at the age of fifty and began drinking. For the rest of his life, he smoked two packs of cigarettes and drank up to two bottles of whiskey a day. The body had been preserved in formaldehyde since death.

Von Hagens wore a blue surgical gown and his trademark black fedora. When a spectator asked whether it was respectful to keep his hat on, von Hagens merely pointed to the surgeon depicted in the reproduction of Rembrandt's "The Anatomy Lesson of Dr. Nicolaes Tulp" which hung above him. He removed the plastic draping the naked and discolored male cadaver. He began the dissection by slicing with a scalpel across the cadaver's hairy chest in a single motion and then perpendicularly from his chest to his stomach, pulling back the flaps of skin with both hands. "The members of audience variously looked away, gasped, covered eyes, gazed in fascination, left the building and at one point applauded" (Cowell 2002). Aesthetically, the autopsy was a sensory experience intended to shock the crowd. The anatomist's actions were mirrored on giant screens inside the gallery, and narrated by pathologist John Lee. The accompanying sounds included what one spectator described as "a general sloshing about of organs" (Cowell 2002), which were passed around in trays after they were removed from the body.

Von Hagens is well-known for inventing the method of preservation he calls "plastination" (discussed above) in which the liquids in the human body are replaced by polymers that make it stable for centuries. With the help of a sizeable staff, von Hagens poses and gas-cures plastinated bodies for display in his five touring BodyWorlds exhibitions. The exhibitions, which have now been seen by 26 million people worldwide, are criticized for making what have been promoted as medical specimens into grotesque sculptures of the dead. Von Hagens appears to thrive on controversy: the media focus on the ethics of his use of human bodies, the questioned origin of some of the corpses, and his strange straddling of art and science only serve to draw more patrons to BodyWorlds. As proprietor of the exhibits, von Hagens — a self-professed showman — is all too happy to be the subject of the attention, and tends to stir up rather than quell controversy. True to form, his announcement that he would conduct a public autopsy provoked the legal and religious authorities, ensuring a sold-out show and an audience more eager for entertainment than the education that the autopsy purported to provide.

Officials allowed the autopsy to take place even though the procedure had not been properly licensed under the 1984 Anatomy Act and was therefore a criminal offense punishable by a three-month jail term. The official Inspector of Anatomy, Dr. Jeremy Metters, explained that a license is required for both the practitioner of a dissection and for the premises in which it is conducted. He had written to von Hagens warning that he faced criminal penalties and that police had been asked to take "appropriate action." Two plainclothes police officers, accompanied by professors of anatomy, took their places in the audience to determine whether the anatomist should be arrested, according to a spokesman for Scotland Yard. Officials had refused to say whether they would stop the autopsy before a crowd and a TV camera crew, but told journalists that a report would be sent to the Crown Prosecution Service to determine whether legal action should be taken (Cowell 2002). But Dr. von Hagens — who seemed to deliberately violate British taboos and sensibilities (Jesperson et al. 2009) — was not worried. Before the autopsy began, he had declared, "I stand here for democracy. This is a democratic country, and I am sure there will be no arrest." In fact, von Hagens had called the event an "autopsy" rather than a "dissection" to skirt the language of the law. Author Helen MacDonald (2005) points out that the cause of death was already known and a death certificate issued.

As they have done regarding his exhibits of plastinated bodies, others questioned the source and legitimacy of the donor body. Originally, von Hagens had planned to carry out his dissection on the body of a 33-year-old epileptic woman, but changed his plan under reported pressure from epilepsy organizations. Instead, the anatomist selected a man who had donated his own body for this purpose, and produced written statements from deceased to prove it. The body donor was aware of the specific use to which his corpse would be put, and had also agreed to plastination of his remains. The autopsied body was subsequently plastinated for display at the BodyWorlds exhibition that opened in Singapore on November 9, 2003. In addition to the donor's written consent, the autopsy was endorsed by the donor's daughter-in-law on television the day it occurred, and sanctioned publicly by his son the following day (Nunn 2005).

The same night as the two-hour live autopsy, a taped version — edited to thirty minutes and supplemented by expert commentary — was broadcast to television viewers of the U.K.'s Channel 4 at 11:45 P.M. in the interest of "demystifying the taboos" that surround death. "It is something that we must all face, yet death has been removed from our normal experience to be managed by professionals," said Simon Andreae, the broadcast's head of science and education (Cowell 2002). Proponents of the autopsy and its televised broadcast thought it only fair that the public understand a procedure that can be conducted by authorities on their own bodies or the bodies of their loved ones after death without consent. The pathologist who participated in the event expressed hope that it would reduce the public's fear and defensiveness about autopsy and organ donation. And in an essay that appears in the companion volume to von Hagens' BodyWorlds exhibitions, Franz Jozef Wetz (2004a) points out a seeming irony: "[I]t would be difficult to make medical laypersons understand why they should be barred from taking part in an autopsy while museums of medical history and the Body Worlds exhibition are readily open for them to visit." True enough, but in a critical essay Christine Jesperson et al. (2009) point out that the dissection and preparation of von Hagens' plastinates is done in secrecy.

Cultural critics and medical ethicists found the claims to substantiate the autopsy dubious. If its measure was to stir talk, headlines, and television chatter around the personage of Gunther von Hagens, then it could be considered a success. It was heavy on sensationalism, with a limited educational aspect that did not justify the degrading and disrespectful way in which it was done (Cowell 2002). Robert Baker, a medical doctor, reflected the views of some members of the audience in calling the spectacle "a travesty of medical science, a grotesque pastiche of a dark but necessary side of the healer's art. What," he asked in a newspaper column, "will be demystified by viewing the performance that couldn't be achieved by looking in a medical encyclopedia or a trip to the butcher?" (Cowell 2002). Michael Wilkes, the head of the British Medical Association's ethics committee, conceded that the "entertainment value was pretty high for some people, with possibly some educational value as well." So, although some dismissed the autopsy as without merit, some people in the audience said afterward that they liked what they saw.

4. Anatomists as Superlatives and Showmen (Gunther von Hagens)

Von Hagens features one adherent in the BodyWorlds companion volume who believes strongly that the lay public should have ready access to the dissection of the human body — to decide for themselves whether or not they benefit from the experience. Wetz (2004a) writes, "... Gunther von Hagens ... is returning to its proper place the thoroughly acceptable, human need to be curious about our anatomy and to feel a pleasant sensation of horror, a sense of awe, and a humble awareness of ourselves as vulnerable, mortal, insignificant creatures. To venture a glance into an unknown body is virtually the same as to discover our own body therein, as only that which can be uncovered and dissected can be comprehended. There is certainly nothing ethically reprehensible in this." Wetz states that he was more horrified by the media frenzy than by the autopsy itself. He describes how the sobriety of the operators, their dispassionate explanations, and the quiet calm in the auditorium "stood in such stark contrast to the heated, often emotional and grim debate conducted in the media and in the public about this demonstration both before and after it took place" (Wetz 2004a). In his opinion, public access should be a right in liberal democracies with an open society, and should be limited only by facility and staffing issues.

In the *Journal of Medical Ethics,* A. Miah (2004) makes clear her belief that the public should be able to experience such events, but questions von Hagens' style. She calls analogies to dissectors of the past, which von Hagens encourages by wearing the now-familiar black fedora, inappropriate. He is not recreating the events of the past, but placing the public autopsy in the new context of the present, a time when privacy and the dignity of the human body are differently understood. Whether the event was "ethical" depends on our cultural interpretation of the body and the concepts associated with it. The fact that autopsies tend not to be public is a product of a particular historical contingency, Miah explains, rather than something ethically or morally absolute. What is more to the point is whether the autopsy was carried out legally, with consent, and in a medically professional manner.

Miah (2004) notes that the public autopsy avoided the rhetoric about aesthetics that the BodyWorlds exhibits provokes, but raises the question of whether it was an appropriate use of a corpse. The assumption is that if the autopsy failed to promote education, it was merely a spectacle and poor use of a human cadaver. The public autopsy's educational value was not merely in trying to show anatomy, but also to demonstrate how inadequately medicine is understood by the public and to challenge the way medicine creates boundaries between public and private. But was this achieved? Miah points out that the TV broadcast focused more on audience reaction than the autopsy itself, and calls the educational aim "marginal." The audience's unease, demonstrated by spontaneous and awkward applause, underlined the sensationalism of the event," she writes (Miah 2004). It seems that von Hagens' event was less about a public autopsy and more about the publicity of an autopsy—an autopsy that he *performed*, in more than one sense of the word.

Von Hagens' autopsy was preceded decades earlier by an avant garde film (since uploaded to YouTube) called "The Act of Seeing with One's Own Eyes" by American experimental filmmaker Stan Brakhage, in which he documented dissection in a Pittsburgh morgue (Jesperson et al. 2009). But his live public dissection has paved the way for a number of media events. Not only have animals (a shark, a squid, and an elephant, for instance) been publicly dissected to benefit museums, but human bodies have been partially autopsied on TV documentaries, notably "Eat to Save Your Life" with British celebrity chef Jamie Oliver and an episode of the American series "The Doctors," which both find additional audiences on YouTube. Then in December 2009, individuals from around the world were welcome to observe a live partial dissection in an institutional context. At the University of California, San Diego Brain Observatory, the frozen brain of Henry Molaison was shaved into thin slices by a microtome. Molaison had died at the age of 82 and his brain was of great interest to researchers. Some of his brain tissue was removed in experimental surgery in 1953 to relieve seizures and he was afterward unable to form memories. He was studied by a neuroscientist for the next fifty years, so there are decades of behavioral data to correlate with the scans that are detailed down to the neurons. Like von Hagens' autopsy, these productions seem to be received as opportunities to indulge morbid interest because of an overpromoted didactic element.

Conclusion

For centuries, the American, British, and European public had the occasional opportunity to watch a corpse being dissected. For large spans of that time, the corpse under the anatomist's knife was an executed felon. Since public dissection was a sanctioned or symbolic supplemental punishment for the capital crime — a combination of physical revenge and spiritual retaliation, the dissector was the agent who meted out that punishment. So not only was dissection associated with the death penalty, the anatomist was seen as an extension of the executioner. He took judicial killing to the next step and, aside from the religious implications, progressively destroyed the body. But to do that, he first had to procure it. His guild or institution may have been on the receiving end of a periodic royal allotment or he may have taken a more proactive approach by vying with others at the foot of the gallows, striking deals with the living for the use of their bodies after death, or haggling with bodysnatchers for the surreptitiously exhumed bodies of the recent dead. This last means of obtaining a subject for his already gruesome demonstrations secured a reputation for the anatomist that lingers to this day. Was not German anatomist Gunther von Hagens repeatedly questioned about the source of the body he dissected publicly in 2002, despite his declaration that it was donated by a man who knew exactly its intended use?

Much of our mistrust of anatomists stems from a long history of questioning their motives. "Why are they so intrigued by carving up the body?" the lay public has wondered, while at the same time shelling out money for tickets to see just that. Their profession has been thought of as a death cult that derives cannibalistic and necrophiliac power from the violation of the dead (Sappol 2002). In practical terms, we worry that they practice indignities on the corpse and, in particular, indecencies upon the dead bodies

Conclusion

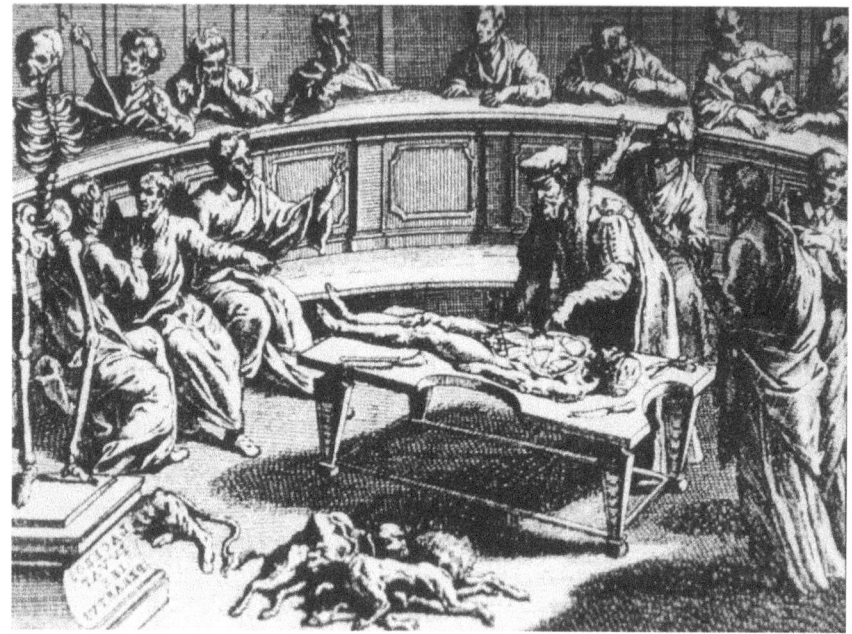

In this interior view of an anatomical theater, a surgeon is examining the cadaver, while men seated and standing observe. An articulated skeleton stands to the left. The copper engraving appeared in Lancisi's edition of the Eustachian plates, 1714 (*courtesy National Library of Medicine*).

of women. As Cuvier's eagerness to spread the legs of the Hottentot Venus after death showed, anatomists looked upon the bodies of others as their own, to do with what they wished. Modest during life, Saartjie Bjartmaan was a genital apron in a specimen jar shortly after it was over. Many a skeleton was harvested from a cadaver, and the skin of an executed prisoner was readily sent to the tannery to be made into bookbindings and souvenirs. After judges were prohibited from sentencing criminals to public dissection, anatomists preyed on the poor instead. In the U.S., they concentrated their bodysnatching on African Americans, whose remains were also accepted as postmortem payment for their medical treatment. Such diabolical deals fed into the long-held belief that anatomy was a godless science — despite attempts by anatomists to use public dissection as an opportunity to demonstrate the hand of God in the ingenious design of the human body.

Conclusion

As they battled superstitions and misperceptions about their dabbling in corpses, anatomists slowly improved their image as a whole. The surgeons of London broke away from the Guild of Barber-Surgeons to form their own company in 1745 and in 1800 received a charter from the throne to become the Royal College of Surgeons of England. They received another boost when the passage of the second Anatomy Act relieved them as agents of the Crown in carrying out the second half of the sentence for notorious crimes — even though this meant one less source of bodies to dissect. They were, however, still closely tied to the bodysnatchers. As the notorious Dr. Knox — who had purchased the victims of Burke and Hare — well knew, disclosures about what happened in dissecting rooms must always shock the public and be hurtful to science (MacDonald 2005). When the bodysnatching scandals disappeared from public consciousness, anatomical dissection disappeared from public gaze. The anatomists withdrew behind the doors of educational institutions, and the townspeople were not invited to join them. No longer associated with execution, dissection was now a scientific pursuit rather than a punishment and was no longer a public performance (MacDonald 2005). Not only that, dissection was not an end in itself anymore, but a stepping stone to related disciplines like pathology. Anatomists had succeeded in specializing and had almost gained the respectability of their longtime rivals, the physicians. The universities realized that surgeons in training needed more practical experience than could be gained at public dissections, and valued that training more highly than polishing stage presence or perpetuating tradition.

Anatomy ended a long history of public performance during which Europeans had erected anatomy theaters modeled after the dramatic theaters of the day and had staged dissections marked by elaborate ceremonies, seating arrangements, ticketed audiences, and the occasional guest anatomist. Even audience members who did not understand Latin were sure to be fascinated by the combination of scientific aura, moral lesson, and morbid entertainment. Vesalius' style is described as "grandiose" and he dissected with dignity and discipline, while keeping his audience captivated. William Harvey, whose public dissections had a political role in continuing to exert control over the surgeons, nevertheless attempted to elicit laughter from his audience. Alexander Monro primus gave lively demonstrations on cadavers he enhanced for the audience by adding color to accentuate the area of focus. Anatomists liked to demonstrate their talents, particularly to well-known and important people whose names they could cite in the textbooks they wrote. But in time it was only those textbooks to which the lay public had access, and the props in the anatomists' stage performances were models rather than authentic bodies. Attitudes had changed and the public distanced themselves from death the same way anatomists had put doors between laypeople and the cadavers they continued to dissect. Mummy unrollings, too — over which reputations had once been won and lost — were a thing of the past. And publicly anatomizing the body of Joice Heth was just an excuse for P.T. Barnum to pull in one last crowd to see "the greatest national and natural curiosity in the world."

The public does still have a morbid curiosity, which brings patrons to the static exhibits in the world's medical museums to see the bottled body parts, the occasional mummy, and the teratology specimens prepared by long-dead anatomists who may have wowed the crowds of their day with live dissections. What Gunther von Hagens knew at the turn of the twenty-first century is that there is still an appetite for the anatomical performance, but few people willing to go up against the legal system and the cultural critics to prove it. Having more than just tested the waters with his circulating BodyWorlds exhibits — populated with oxymoronically dynamic still lifes, he used one of his designated donor bodies to show a select audience exactly how he breaches the corpse's exterior to prepare an anatomical figure. He stood before them, scalpel in hand, to demonstrate the "Y-incision" they had probably seen many times on crime dramas, but never in person. He split the ribcage and removed the organs, which the audience members may also have seen on television. And then he sent one of those organs into the seats on a tray, which was likely a first for many. This gesture reinforced the idea that they were *participants* in this resurrection of a historic pastime. They were not grabbing at the scraps like some of their less well-behaved forbears, and there were classical anatomical artworks on the walls rather than damask decorations. The show was secular, medical, and rather than showing the wondrous creation that is the human body, von Hagens was revealing what a lifetime of smoking and drinking will do to the liver and lungs.

Conclusion

In the early public demonstration of anatomy, the dissector strove to astound the audience as he explored the body to tell a moral tale rather different than the consequences of bad behavior. He meant the audience to marvel at the intricacies of the wondrous creation of God and to be awed by the interconnected parts his scalpel made visible to them. The dissection was a show with religious overtones and to witness it was to greater appreciate God's design. Later, when the cadaver on the table was an executed felon, the dissection conveyed a different lesson, that of just desserts, in which the subject is exposed in every sense of the word as part of the punishment for criminal acts. By the time von Hagens performed his public demonstration, it had been centuries since dissections had had a religious or a punitive connotation. It was the question of ethics that was raised, since the remaining reason for the event — beyond the thin veneer of medical education — was entertainment. And this motivator has its own long history. At the institutional dissections to which the public was admitted, the students were there to observe and learn from a task which they may in the future perform themselves, while the other visitors were either inspired by a desire to educate themselves or drawn merely by the sensation of seeing someone — presumably with showmanship — cut up a cadaver. And it was a show they paid for by purchasing a ticket, so they did not expect to be disappointed, whether they were a Philadelphia audience clamoring for entrance to see the dissection of conjoined twins (Sappol 2002) or a London audience taking their seats to watch an Egyptologist chip away at the hardened coverings that wrapped an ancient corpse, simultaneously "penetrating the mysteries of the ages" (Lyu 2005).

The ideas of observing a dissection to learn from a body and to be entertained by it are not mutually exclusive. They may compete, but both motivations stem from a curiosity about both the outside and the inside of a corpse, and have continued long after religious taboos about dissection were lifted. There have been numerous historical examples of morbid fascination leading crowds to cadavers. As two examples, sightseers toured the Paris morgue by the tens of thousands under the precept of identifying unknown corpses, and in Chicago after the death of John Dillinger in 1934, thousands paraded through the Cook County Morgue to see his body after it was autopsied and thousands more passed by his remains after they were prepared at an Indiana funeral home. This neck-stretching curiosity is not just the prerogative of the public. Doctors, too, have exhibited a lurid interest that exceeds their clinical curiosity. It was more than their interest in comparative anatomy that brought medical and veterinary students to Fragonard's tour de force, the dissected and permanently preserved "Horse and Rider." And more than one hundred years later, a mostly lay audience is drawn to von Hagens' enormous, vivid, and stunning replication of Fragonard's best-known preparation.

Fragonard's standing bodies and galloping horse were ostensibly produced as aesthetically-considered teaching aids. Von Hagens' upright plastinates and rearing stallion are installed in a series of science museums and framed in terms of their anatomical value. As the eighteenth-century French anatomist's motives were questioned by his contemporaries, so has his twenty-first century German counterpart often had to fend off accusations that he is simply sculpting human bodies. But art and anatomy have long been intertwined, in two-dimensional illustrations and in three-dimensional preparations. Some believed that the scientific purposes for creating the anatomical waxes in the 1800s were just an excuse for depicting beautiful, sensual dying women, yet they were also produced to correspond to the poses depicted in medical texts. Von Hagens lifts the flat figures from anatomical atlases into life-size tableaux starring his anonymous plastinates, and in his case it is not just to anatomize and to aestheticize, to symbolize like Susini, or to moralize like Ruysch, but to tout his now twenty-year-old but still premier preservation method. In this way, von Hagens departs from his predecessors, who guarded their embalming formulae carefully. He explains his patented process completely as yet another means of amazing his audience.

This openness sets up a tension between the historical necessity to suppress and the contemporary compulsion to impress (Simon 2002). The sight of so many plastinates and the thrill of watching the plastinator dissect yet one more become spectacle. The active event, especially, is more of a spectacle than the corpse of a villain being cut up to make souvenirs after a hasty hanging or a body being taken apart by candlelight accompanied by Latin recitation. This is because between the eighteenth century and today, death has been medicalized (Simon 2002) and the medical profession has co-opted the corpse, including its dissection. This

Conclusion

goes beyond the ethical argument that von Hagens is flaunting the privacy and the dignity of the human body, concepts which are differently understood today than they were in previous centuries (Miah 2004). There is the idea that he has betrayed his medical credentials by "outing" the dissected cadaver. Von Hagens did so first by presenting static écorchés and then, when he promoted and performed his public autopsy in 2002, as live spectacle. Delivered under what colleagues and critics considered the *guise* of bringing anatomical knowledge directly to the public, the anatomist provoked questions about propriety and morbid curiosity that we thought we had put behind us. Von Hagens raises the question of whether observing dissection should be exclusive to medical education, despite differences in public sentiment about the dead body in our own age. And he does not just ask, he puts it to the test. But if the anatomists of the past had not simply forged ahead, would the discipline have advanced?

The history of anatomy shows patterns of continuity, despite societal differences, punctuated by revolutionaries like Vesalius and showmen (show-offs?) like Fragonard. Sons followed in the footsteps of their fathers, for instance Edinburgh's three-generation Monro dynasty, and students followed where their well-known mentors left off. Pupils were instructed, textbooks were illustrated, specimens were collected and preserved. Anatomists no longer haggle with the hangman beneath the noose and they no longer harvest the hide of cadavers to rebind their medical books, because laws and minds have changed. They do, however, emulate their predecessors in ways the layperson may find difficult to understand. It made the international news when an anatomist from India dissected his father in 2010, as English physician William Harvey had four hundred years earlier. Fragonard's ambition in the 1700s was to create a virtual cadaver factory in which to produce a great number of specimens, a dream that von Hagens has fulfilled in our day and age by employing a staff of dozens to produce plastinates under his direction.

Unlike many anatomists over the years, who have taken pains to ensure that their bodies did not go under the knife posthumously, Gunther von Hagens has made it his stated intention to be dissected, plastinated, posed, and put on display. The announcement of this decision may have been self-serving, succeeding in keeping his name in the news, as it has been during his many other controversies. Not least of the publicity-garnering revelations was his announcement that he would perform a live dissection before an audience. But it is the definition of dissection to *demonstrate*, and von Hagens has taken up the mantle of showing anatomy to the paying public. He relishes comparison with the anatomists of the past, even though some may feel that he is more aptly compared to fellow showman P.T. Barnum. But this, too, has precedent, and from early on in the discipline. Biographer Wendy Moore (2005) calls second-century surgeon Galen "an irrepressible showman, like so many anatomists down the centuries." Opposite the quietly industrious and often unnamed anatomists who toiled alongside the wax artisans and lent their expertise to textbooks illustrators and anatomical model-makers were performers like William Harvey, who liked to keep his audience amused as he explained the intricacies of the dissected cadaver that lay before him.

Except for the few hundred at von Hagen's public dissection, the audiences of today's anatomical demonstrations are standing in the secure laboratories of medical schools rather than set squarely in the midst of common culture. In the modern era, the anatomist is rarely the subject of a famous painting like Doctors Deyman, Ruysch, and Tulp. The demonstrator is more often a figure hovering on the periphery of an informal class photograph posed in the dissection room. In the twenty-first century, even that is no longer allowed for fear that the images will leak out and spoil the privacy of the body donor or soil the reputation of the anatomy department, which already carries with it so much historical baggage. The discipline of anatomy, not so much the mechanics of dissection, has changed. And the uninitiated audience is relatively unaware of the long tradition that leads from Herophilus in the third century through Mondino de Liuzzi in the fourteenth century to von Hagens in our own. Remember that when a member of his audience asked whether it was respectful to keep his black hat on during the dissection, von Hagens simply gestured toward his predecessor Dr. Tulp in the Rembrandt reproduction that hung over his head. Dr. Tulp had in fact patterned himself after Vesalius. History shows that Dr. Gunther von Hagens comes by his dramatic flourishes and self-promotion naturally. Like Vesalius in the sixteenth century and Ruysch in the eighteenth, von Hagens will be remembered as the great anatomist of his age. And with that, we avert our eyes from what's left of the corpse and exit the anatomy theater.

Bibliography

Angel, Maria. 2004. "Physiology and Fabrication: The Art of Making Visible." In Elizabeth Klaver, ed., *Images of the Corpse: From the Renaissance to Cyberspace*. Madison: University of Wisconsin Press.

"Archæologica Medica XLV: William Cheselden, Anatomist And Surgeon." 1898. *The British Medical Journal* Vol. 2, No. 1968 (Sept. 17): 815–817.

Ariès, Philippe. 1982. *The Hour of Our Death*. New York: Vintage.

Arnold, Eugene A. 2004. "Autopsy: The Final Diagnosis." In Elizabeth Klaver, ed., *Images of the Corpse: From the Renaissance to Cyberspace*. Madison: University of Wisconsin Press.

Baljet, B. 2000. "The Painted Amsterdam Anatomy Lessons: Anatomy Performances in Dissecting Rooms?" *Annals of Anatomy* Vol. 182, No. 1 (Jan.): 3–11.

Ballestriero, Robert. 2010. "Anatomical Models and Wax Venuses: Art Masterpieces or Scientific Craft Works?" *Journal of Anatomy* Vol. 216, No. 2 (Feb.): 223–234.

Barker, Francis. 1984. *The Tremulous Private Body: Essays on Subjection*. London: Methuen.

Barnum, Phineas Taylor. 1888. *The Life of P.T. Barnum, Written by Himself, including his Golden Rules for Money-Making*. Buffalo: The Courier Co. [http://books.google.com/books?id=aVQPsBciUswC&printsec=frontcover#v=onepage&q&f=false, accessed 6/20/2010].

Bauer, Axel W. 2004. "Plastinated Specimens and their Presentation in Museums: A Theoretical and Bioethical Retrospective on a Media Event." In Gunther von Hagens and Angelina Whalley, *Body Worlds: The Anatomical Exhibition of Real Human Bodies*. Heidelberg: Institut für Plastination.

Baumgarten, Elias. 2001. "Curiosity as a Moral Virtue." *International Journal of Applied Philosophy* (Fall).

Berger, John. 1972. *Ways of Seeing*. London: BBC and Penguin.

"BodyWorlds Creator, Anatomist Gunther von Hagens Reveals His Two Year Life-Changing Battle with Parkinson's Disease." 2010. *PR Newswire* (Dec. 29) [http://www.prnewswire.com/news-releases/body-worlds-creator-anatomist-gunther-von-hagens-reveals-his-two-year-life-changing-battle-with-parkinsons-disease-112603869.html, accessed 1/24/11].

Bohannon, John, Ding Yimin, and Xiong Lei. 2003. "Anatomy's Full Monty." *Science* Vol. 301 (Aug. 29): 5637.

Bolter, Jay David, and Richard Grusin. 1998. *Remediation: Understanding New Media*. Cambridge: MIT Press.

Bradbury, Mary. 1999. *Representations of Death: A Social Psychological Perspective*. New York: Routledge.

Brock, Bazon. 2004. "The Educating Power of the Sciences." In Gunther von Hagens and Angelina Whalley, *Body Worlds: The Anatomical Exhibition of Real Human Bodies*. Heidelberg: Institut für Plastination.

Burton, John W. 2001. *Culture and the Human Body*. Propect Heights, IL: Waveland Press.

Carlino, Andrea. 1999. *Books of the Body: Anatomical Ritual and Renaissance Learning*. Translated by John Tedeschi and Anne C. Tedeschi. Chicago: University of Chicago Press.

Carpenter, Lucas. 2001. "London, England." *Art Papers* Vol. 26, No. 6: 58.

"Clemente Susini's Wax Anatomical Models at the University of Cagliari." 2002. Cagliari, Italy: Università di Cagliari [http://pacs.unica.it/cere/mono03_en.htm, accessed 8/20/2011].

Cockburn, A., E. Cockburn, and T.A. Reyman. 1998. *Mummies, Disease & Ancient Cultures, 2nd Edition*. Cambridge: Cambridge University Press.

Cooper, Bransby Blake. 1843. *The Life of Sir Astley Cooper, Bart., Interspersed with Sketches from his Note-Books of Distinguished Contemporary Characters*. London: John W. Parker [http://books.google.com/books?id=AwQLAAAAYAAJ&pg=PR20&dq=sir+astley+cooper&hl=en&ei=h6d9TLWpCoK88gb98JjnBg&sa=X&oi=book_result&ct=result&resnum=7&ved=0CEgQ6AEwBg#v=onepage&q&f=false , accessed 8/31/10, 6/24/11].

Cowell, Alan. 2002. "Art or Ghoulishness? Autopsy is TV Spectacle in Britain." *The New York Times* (Nov. 22) [http://www.nytimes.com/2002/11/22/world/art-or-ghoulishness-autopsy-is-tv-spectacle-in-britain.html?scp=1&sq=art%20or%20ghoulishness?%20autopsy%20is%20TV%20spectacle%20in%20britain&st=cse, accessed 5/4/10].

Cregan, Kate. 2004. "Blood and Circuses." In Elizabeth Klaver, ed., *Images of the Corpse: From the Renaissance to Cyberspace*. Madison: University of Wisconsin Press.

Csikszentmihalyi, Mihalyi, and Rick E. Robinson. 1990. *The Art of Seeing: An Interpretation of the Aesthetic Experience*. Malibu: J. Paul Getty Trust Fund.

Dawson, Warren R. 1934. "Pettigrew's Demonstrations upon Mummies: A Chapter in the History of Egyptology." The Journal of Egyptian Archaeology Vol. 20, No. 3/4 (Nov.): 170–182 [http://www.jstor.org/stable/3854736, accessed 5/19/09].

de Ceglia, Francesco Paolo. 2005. "The Rotten, the Disembowelled Woman, the Skinned Man: Body Images from Eighteenth century Florentine Wax Modelling." *Journal of Science Communication* Vol. 4, No. 3 (Oct.).

Douglas, Mary. 1996. "The Two Bodies." *Natural Symbols*. London: Routledge.

Downs, Robert D. 2004. *Books That Changed the World*. New York: Signet.

Driessen van het Reve, Jozien J., and Anna B. Radzyun. n.d. "The Anatomical

Preparations of Frederik Ruysch." Amsterdam, The Netherlands: Universiteit van Amsterdam [http://ruysch.dpc.uba.uva.nl/cgi/t/text/text-idx?c=ruysch;lang=en;page=home, accessed 9/1/2011].

Dunand, F., and R. Lichtenberg. 2006. *Mummies and Death in Egypt*. Translated by D. Lorton. Ithaca, New York: Cornell University Press.

Edwards, Linden F. 1955. *Cincinnati's "Old Cunny": A Notorious Purveyor of Human Flesh*. Fort Wayne, IN: Public Library of Fort Wayne and Allen County.

El Mahdy, C. 1989. *Mummies, Myth and Magic in Ancient Egypt*. London: Thames & Hudson.

Erlanger, Steven. 2011. "Exhibitor of Bodies Intends to Contribute His Own." *New York Times* (Jan. 5) [http://www.nytimes.com/2011/01/06/world/europe/06corpses.html?_r=3&ref=todayspaper, accessed 1/11/11].

"Execution of Burke." 1829. *The Scotsman*. Jan. 31 [http://archive.scotsman.com/article.cfm?id=TSC/1829/01/31/Ar00601, accessed 5/11/09].

Ferrari, Giovanna. 1987. "Public Anatomy Lessons and the Carnival: The Anatomy Theatre of Bologna." *Past and Present* No. 117 (Nov.): 50–106.

Finkelstein, David and Alistair McCleary, eds. 2002. *The Book History Reader*. New York: Routledge.

Fischer, Ulrich. 2004. "When Death Goes on Display." In Gunther von Hagens and Angelina Whalley, *Body Worlds: The Anatomical Exhibition of Real Human Bodies*. Heidelberg: Institut für Plastination.

Fitzpatrick, Michael. 2002. "Making a Spectacle of Ourselves." *Spiked* Mar. 26.

Flatt, Adrian E. 2009. "Happy Birthday, *Gray's Anatomy!*" *Baylor University Medical Center Proceedings* Vol. 22, No. 4 (Oct.): 342–345 [http://www.ncbi.nlm.nih.gov/pmc/articles/PMC2760169/, accessed 8/6/11].

Foot, Mirjam. 1993. "Bookbinding and the History of Books." In Nicholas Barker, ed., *A Potencie of Life: Books in Society*. London: British Library.

French, Roger. 1999. *Dissection and Vivisection in the European Renaissance*. Aldershot, England: Ashgate.

Gairdner, John. 1860. *Historical Sketch of the Royal College of Surgeons of Edinburgh; Being an Address Delivered on 19th January 1860, at a Conversazione in a Hall of the College; With Notes and Documents*. Edinburgh: Sutherland and Knox [http://books.google.com/books?id=rglbAAAAQAAJ&printsec=frontcover&dq=Historical+sketch+of+the+Royal+College+of+Surgeons+of+Edinburgh&hl=en&ei=3dtyTPWLKIP98AaQtN3eCw&sa=X&oi=book_result&ct=result&resnum=1&ved=0CCkQ6AEwAA#v=onepage&q&f=false, accessed 8/22/10].

Gonzalez-Crussi, F., and Rosamond Purcell. 1995. *Suspended Animation: Six Essays on the Preservation of Bodily Parts*. San Francisco: Harcourt Brace & Co.

Gould, Stephen Jay. 1982. "The Hottentot Venus." *Natural History* Vol. 91: 20–7.

_____. 1985. *The Flamingo's Smile: Reflections in Natural History*. New York: Norton.

Gould, Stephen Jay, and Rosamond Wolff Purcell. 2000. *Crossing Over: Where Art and Science Meet*. New York: Three Rivers Press.

Gribben, Mark. n.d. "Sweeney Todd." TruTV Crime Library [http://www.trutv.com/library/crime/serial_killers/weird/todd/index_1.html, accessed 5/14/09].

"Gunther von Hagens Exhibition Criticised over Corpse Sex Display." 2009. *The Telegraph* (May 7) [http://www.telegraph.co.uk/news/newstopics/howaboutthat/5289311/Gunther-von-Hagens-exhibition-criticised-over-corpse-sex-display.html, accessed 1/24/11].

Haithman, Diane. 2004. "Anatomy Exhibit in Los Angeles Called Both Gross and Engrossing." *Los Angeles Times* (June 27).

Hallam, Elizabeth, Jenny Hockey, and Glennys Howarth. 1999. *Beyond the Body: Death and Social Identity*. London: Routledge.

Hansen, Julie V. 1996. "Resurrecting Death: Anatomical Art in the Cabinet of Dr. Frederik ARuysch." *The Art Bulletin* Vol. 78, No. 4 (Dec.): 663–679.

Hartmann, George W. 1974. *Gestalt Psychology: A Survey of Facts and Principles*. Westport, CT: Greenwood Press.

Harvey, Doug. 2004. "The Exquisite Corpses of Dr. von Hagens." *LA Weekly* (July 23–29).

Hayes, Bill. 2008. *The Anatomist: A True Story of Gray's Anatomy*. New York: Ballantine.

"He Stands by his Trade: A Bodysnatcher Sells his Own Body." 1878. *New York Times*. Aug. 9 [http://query.nytimes.com/mem/archive-free/pdf?res=F40A14FC3B5C1B7B93CBA91783D85F4C8784F9, accessed 1/9/10].

Heather, Rosemary. 2002. "Gunther von Hagens." *Border Crossings* Vol. 21, No. 3 (Aug.).

Hillman, David, and Carla Mazzio, eds. 1997. *The Body in Parts: Fantasies of Corporeality in Early Modern Europe*. London: Routledge.

Holmes, Rachel. 2007. *African Queen: The Real Life of the Hottentot Venus*. New York: Random House.

Holubar, Karl. 1991. "The Anatomical Wax Preparations in the Josephinum in Vienna, Austria." *Archives of Surgery* Vol. 126 (April): 421–422.

Hooper-Greenhill, Eilean, ed. 1994. *The Educational Role of the Museum*. New York: Routledge.

Hopwood, Nick. 2008. "The Art of Medicine: Model Politics." *The Lancet* Vol. 372 (Dec. 6): 1946.

Hove, L.M., S. Young, and J.C. Schrama. 2008. "Dr. Nicolaes Tulp's Anatomy Lecture." *The Journal of the Norwegian Medical Association* Vol. 128: 716–9 [http://www.tidsskriftet.no/index.php?seks_id_eng=37670&seks_id=1667756, accessed 9/27/10].

Ikram, S., and A. Dodson. 1998. *The Mummy in Ancient Egypt*. London: Thames & Hudson.

Infusino, Mark H., Dorothy Win, and Ynez V. O'Neill. 1995. "Mondino's Book and the Human Body." *Vesalius* Vol. 1, No. 2: 71–76.

Jackson, Holbrook. 1932. "Books Bound in Human Skin." *The Anatomy of Bibliomania*. New York: Charles Scribner's Sons.

Jeffries, Stuart. 2002. "The Naked and the Dead." *The Guardian* (Mar. 19).

Jespersen, T. Christine, Alicita Rodríguez, and Joseph Starr, eds. 2009. *The Anatomy of Body Worlds: Critical Essays on the Plastinated Cadavers of Gunther von Hagens*. Jefferson, NC: McFarland.
Johnson, Stephen. 2009. "The Persistence of Tradition in Anatomical Museums." In T. Christine Jesperson et al., eds., *The Anatomy of BodyWorlds*. Jefferson, NC: McFarland.
Jones, D. G. 2002. "Re-inventing Anatomy: The Impact of Plastination on How We See the Human Body." *Clinical Anatomy* Vol. 15: 436–440.
Karp, Ivan, and Steven D. Lavine, eds. 1991. *Exhibiting Cultures: The Poetics and Politics of Museum Display*. Washington, DC: Smithsonian Institution Press.
Katz, David. 1979. *Gestalt Psychology: Its Nature and Significance*. Westport, CT: Greenwood Press.
Kemp, Martin. 2010. "Style and Non-Style in Anatomical illustration: From Renaissance Humanism to Henry Gray." *Journal of Anatomy* Vol. 216: 192–208.
Kemp, Martin, and Marina Wallace. 2000. *Spectacular Bodies: The Art and Science of the Human Body from Leonardo to Now*. London: Hayward Gallery.
Klaver, Elizabeth, ed. 2004. *Images of the Corpse: From the Renaissance to Cyberspace*. Madison: University of Wisconsin Press.
Kleinschmidt, Nina, and Henri Wagner. 2000. *Endlich Unsterblich? Gunther von Hagens — Schöpfer der Körperwelten*. Band: Bastei Lübbe.
Klestinec C. 2006. "Vesalius and the Print Culture: Public Dissection as Intimate Ritual." *Konteksty—Polska Sztuka Ludowa (Polish Folk Art—Contexts)* Vol. 60, No. 1: 15–25 [http://cejsh.icm.edu.pl/cejsh/cgi-bin/getdoc.cgi?07PLAAAA021 64553, accessed 6/22/09].
Knipfel, Jim. 1998. "Body Art: What a Piece of Work." *New York Press* Vol. 11, No. 26 (July 1–7): 34–35.
Kobler, John. 1988. *The Reluctant Surgeon: A Biography of John Hunter*. Pleasantville, NY: Akadine Press.
Kress, Gunther, and Theo van Leeuwen. 1996. *Reading Images: The Grammar of Visual Design*. London: Routledge.
Kristeva, Julia. 1982. *Powers of Horror: An Essay on Abjection*. New York: Columbia University Press.
Kriz, Wilhelm. 2004. "Foreword." In Gunther von Hagens and Angelina Whalley, *Body Worlds: The Anatomical Exhibition of Real Human Bodies*. Heidelberg: Institut für Plastination.
"Kunstkamera: Peter the Great Museum of Anthropology and Ethnology." n.d. [http://www.kunstkamera.ru/en/, accessed 9/2/2011].
"Lady Gaga to bring bodies on stage." 2010. *Sify News* (June 23) [http://www.sify.com/news/lady-gaga-to-bring-bodies-on-stage-news-international-kgxvkpcbghc.html, accessed 1/24/11].
Landler, Mark. 2004. "A New Spine-Tingler from the Impresario of Cadavers." *New York Times* (Feb. 3).
Lantermann, Ernst-D. 2004. "Körperwelten as Seen by Visitors: Visitor Survey Report from the First Exhibition in Europe." In Gunther von Hagens and

Angelina Whalley, *Body Worlds: The Anatomical Exhibition of Real Human Bodies.* Heidelberg: Institut für Plastination.

Lara, Adair. 2005. "Seeing Dead People." *The San Francisco Chronicle* (Mar. 27).

Lassek, Arthur M. 1958. *Human Dissection: Its Drama and Struggle.* Springfield, IL: C.C. Thomas [http://www.archive.org/details/humandissectioni00lassrich, accessed 5/28/2010].

Laurence, John. 1963. *A History of Capital Punishment.* New York: Citadel Press.

Leder, Drew. 1992. "A Tale of Two Bodies: The Cartesian Corpse and the Lived Body." In Drew Leder, ed. *The Body in Medical Thought and Practice.* Dordrecht: Kluwer Academic Publishers.

———, ed. 1992. *The Body in Medical Thought and Practice.* Dordrecht: Kluwer Academic Publishers.

Lemire, M. 1992. "Representation of the Human Body: The Colored Wax Anatomic Models of the Eighteenth and Nineteenth Centuries in the Revival of Medical Instruction." *Journal of Clinical Anatomy* Vol. 14: 283–291.

The Life of Joice Heth, the Nurse of Gen. George Washington, (the Father of Our Country,) Now Living at the Astonishing Age of 161 Years, and Weighs Only 46 Pounds. 1835. New York [http://docsouth.unc.edu/neh/heth/heth.html, accessed 6/20/2010].

Luyendijk-Elshout, Antonie M. 1970. "Death Enlightened: A Study of Frederik Ruysch." *Journal of the American Medical Association* Vol. 212, No. 1 (April 6): 121–126.

Lyu, Claire. 2005. "Unswathing the Mummy: Body, Knowledge, and Writing in Gautier's *Le Roman de la momie.*" *Nineteenth Century French Studies* Vol. 33, No. 3 and 4: 308–319.

MacDonald, Helen. 2005. *Human Remains: Dissection and Its Histories.* New Haven, CT: Yale University Press.

Malomo, A.O., O.E. Idowu, and F.C. Osuagwu. 2006. "Lessons from History: Human Anatomy, from the Origin to the Renaissance." *International Journal of Morphology* Vol. 24, No. 1: 99–104.

Message, Kylie Rachel. 2004. "Watching Over the Wounded Eyes of Georges Bataille and Andres Serrano." In Elizabeth Klaver, ed., *Images of the Corpse: From the Renaissance to Cyberspace.* Madison: University of Wisconsin Press.

Messbarger, Rebecca. 2010. *The Lady Anatomist: The Life and Work of Anna Morandi Manzolini.* Chicago: University of Chicago Press.

Miah, A. 2004. "The Public Autopsy: Somewhere Between Art, Education, and Entertainment." *Journal of Medical Ethics* Vol. 30: 576–579.

Mirilas, Petros, Panagiotis Lainas, Dimitrios Panutsopulos, Panagiotis N. Skandalakis, and John E. Skandalakis. 2006. "The Monarch and the Master: Peter the Great and Frederik Ruysch." *Archives of Surgery,* Vol. 141 (June): 602–606.

Montross, Christine. 2007. *Body of Work.* New York: Penguin Press.

Mooallem, Jon. 2005. "I See Dead People." Salon.com (June 5).

Moore, Charleen M., and C. Mackenzie Brown. 2004. "Gunther von Hagens and Body Worlds, Part 1: The Anatomist as Prosektor and Proplastiker." In Gunther von Hagens and Angelina Whalley, *Body Worlds: The Anatomical Exhibition of Real Human Bodies*. Heidelberg: Institut für Plastination.

_____, and _____. 2004. "Gunther von Hagens and Body Worlds, Part 2: The Anatomist as Priest and Prophet." In Gunther von Hagens and Angelina Whalley, *Body Worlds: The Anatomical Exhibition of Real Human Bodies*. Heidelberg: Institut für Plastination.

Moore, Wendy. 2005. *The Knife Man: Blood, Body Snatching, and the Birth of Surgery*. New York: Broadway.

Morris, Richard. 2002. "Public Dissection: Press Release." Horsham District Council (Nov. 10) [http://www.horsham.gov.uk/your_area/News/news_2130.asp, accessed 5/7/2009].

"A Mummy Unrolled: Details of an Interesting Exhibition in London." 1889. *The New York Times* (Dec. 30) [http://query.nytimes.com/mem/archive-free/pdf?_r=3&res=9E06E2D7133AE033A25753C3A9649D94689FD7CF&oref=slogin, accessed 5/18/09].

"Museo dello Cere Anatomiche 'Luigi Cattaneo.'" n.d. [www.museocereanatomiche.it, accessed 8/19/2011].

Neher, Allister. 2010. "The Truth about Our Bones: William Cheselden's *Osteographia*." *Medical History* Vol. 54: 517–528.

Norfleet, Barbara P. 1993. *Looking at Death*. Boston: David R. Godine.

Nunn, Hillary. 2005. *Staging Anatomies: Dissection and Spectacle in Early Stuart Tragedy* (Aldershot, England: Ashgate).

Oliver, Jamie. 2008. "Eat to Save Your Life" [http://www.youtube.com/watch?v=JXLRnpS0oCI (6:40) and http://www.youtube.com/watch?v=rcgOwv-L24Y&NR=1, accessed 6/12/09].

Ong, Walter. 2002. "Orality and Literacy: Writing Restructures Consciousness." In David Finkelstein and Alistair McCleary, eds., *The Book History Reader*. New York: Routledge.

Ore, Mary. 2002. "Anatomy as Art: Unsettling but Drawing Crowds." *New York Times* (July 9).

Padley, Jonathan. 2003. "Frankenstein and (Sublime) Creation." *Romanticism* Vol. 9, No. 2.

Panzanelli, Roberta. 2008. *Ephemeral Bodies: Wax Sculpture and the Human Figure*. Los Angeles: Getty Research Institute.

Park, Katharine. 1994. "The Criminal and the Saintly Body: Autopsy and Dissection in Renaissance Italy." *Renaissance Quarterly* Vol. 47, No. 1 (Spring): 1–33.

Parker, Dewitt H. 2004. *The Principles of Aesthetics*. Project Gutenberg.

Payne, Lynda. 2002. "'With much nausea, loathing, and foetor': William Harvey, dissection, and dispassion in early modern medicine." *Vesalius* Vol. 8, No. 2 (Dec.): 45–52.

Petherbridge, Deanna, and Ludmilla Jordanova. 1997. *The Quick and the Dead: Artists and Anatomy*. Berkeley: University of California Press.

Pierson, Patricia. 2009. "The Amethyst Seal: Anatomy and Identity in Bentham and von Hagens." In T. Christine Jesperson et al., eds., *The Anatomy of Body-Worlds*. Jefferson, NC: McFarland.

Ponce, Pedro. 2009. "Illuminating the Soul: Panopticism and the Freak Show." In T. Christine Jesperson et al., eds., *The Anatomy of BodyWorlds*. Jefferson, NC: McFarland.

Porter, Roy. 1991. "Bodies of Thought: Thoughts about the Body in Eighteenth-Century England." In Joan H. Pittock and Andrew Wear, eds., *Interpretation and Cultural History*. London: Macmillan.

_____. 2003. *Flesh in the Age of Reason*. New York: W.W. Norton.

"The Red Barn Murder." n.d. West Suffolk, England: St. Edmundsbury Borough Council. [http://www.stedmundsbury.gov.uk/sebc/visit/redbarn-intro.cfm, accessed 5/13/2009].

Richardson, Ruth. 1987. *Death, Dissection and the Destitute*. London: Routledge & Kegan Paul.

_____. 2009. *The Making of Mr. Gray's Anatomy: Bodies, Books, Fortune, Fame*. New York: Oxford University Press.

Roberts, K.B., and J.D.W. Tomlinson. 1992. *The Fabric of the Body: European Traditions of Anatomical Illustration*. Oxford: Clarendon Press.

Rowe, Katherine. 1997. "'God's Handy Worke." In David Hillman and Carla Mazzio, eds., *The Body in Parts: Fantasies of Corporeality in Early Modern Europe*. New York: Routledge.

Royal College of Physicians of London, eds. 1886. *Prelectiones Anatomia Universalis by William Harvey*. London: J. & A. Churchill.

Sappol, Michael. 2002. *A Traffic of Dead Bodies: Anatomy and Embodied Racial Identity in Nineteenth-Century America*. Princeton, NJ: Princeton University Press.

_____. 2004. "'Morbid curiosity': The Decline and Fall of the Popular Anatomical Museum." *Common-Place* Vol. 4, No. 2 (Jan.).

Sato, Akiro. 1994. *Anatomia Barocca: Museo Zoologico "La Specola" dell Universita a Firenze*. Tokyo: Treville.

Sawday, Jonathan. 1995. *The Body Emblazoned: Dissection and the Human Body in Renaissance Culture*. London: Routledge.

Schiebinger, Linda. 2000. "Taxonomy for Human Beings." In Gill Kirkup, Linda Janes, Kathryn Woodward, and Fiona Hovenden, eds., *The Gendered Cyborg: A Reader*. London: Routledge.

Schnalke, Thomas. 2004. "Dissected Limbs and the Integral Body: On Anatomical Wax Models and Medical Moulages." *Interdisciplinary Science Reviews* Vol. 29, No. 3 (Sept.): 312–322.

Schumacher, Gert-Horst. 2007. "*Theatrum Anatomicum* in History and Today." *International Journal of Morphology* Vol. 25, No. 1: 15–32 [http://www.scielo.cl/scielo.php?pid=S0717-95022007000100002&script=sci_arttext, accessed 6/6/09].

Scott, Gillian. 2009. Personal communication. July 21.

Searle, Adrian. 2002. "Getting Under the Skin." *The Guardian* (Mar. 23).

Seipel, W. 1996. "Mummies and Ethics in the Museum." In Spindler, K., H. Wilfing, E. Rastbichler-Zissernig, D. zur Nedden, and H. Nothdurfter, Editors. *Human Mummies: A Global Survey of their Status and the Techniques of Conservation.* New York: Springer-Verlag.

Shlain, Leonard. 1991. *Art and Physics: Parallel Visions in Space, Time, and Light.* New York: William Morrow.

Shultz, Suzanne M. 1992. *Body Snatching: The Robbing of Graves for the Education of Physicians in Early Nineteenth Century America.* Jefferson, NC: McFarland.

Simon, Jonathan. 2002. "The Theater of Anatomy: The Anatomical Preparations of Honoré Fragonard." *Eighteenth-Century Studies* Vol. 36, No. 1 (Fall): 63–79.

Singh, Debashis. 2003. "Scientist or Showman?" *British Medical Journal* Vol. 326 (Mar. 1): 468.

Spitzack, Carole. 1992. "Foucault's Political Body in Medical Praxis." In Drew Leder, ed., *The Body in Medical Thought and Practice.* Dordrecht: Kluwer Academic Publishers.

Sturken, Marita, and Lisa Cartwright. 2001. *Practices of Looking: An Introduction to Visual Culture.* Oxford: Oxford University Press.

Synott, A. 1992. "Tomb, Temple, Machine and Self: The Social Construction of the Body." *British Journal of Sociology* Vol. 43, No. 1: 79–110.

van Dijck, José. 2001. "Bodyworlds: The Art of Plastinated Cadavers." *Configurations* Vol. 9: 99–126.

_____. 2005. *The Transparent Body: A Cultural Analysis of Medical Imaging.* Seattle: University of Washington Press.

Von During, Monika, Marta Poggesi, and Georges Didi-Huberman. 1999. *Encyclopaedia Anatomica: Museo La Specola Florence, A Complete Collection of Anatomical Waxes.* Koln, Germany: Taschen.

von Hagens, Gunther. 2004a. "Anatomy and Plastination." In Gunther von Hagens and Angelina Whalley, *Body Worlds: The Anatomical Exhibition of Real Human Bodies.* Heidelberg: Institut für Plastination.

_____. 2004b. "On Gruesome Corpses, Gestalt Plastinates and Mandatory Interment." In Gunther von Hagens and Angelina Whalley, *Body Worlds: The Anatomical Exhibition of Real Human Bodies.* Heidelberg: Institut für Plastination.

von Hagens, Gunther, and Angelina Whalley. 2004. *Body Worlds: The Anatomical Exhibition of Real Human Bodies.* Heidelberg: Institut für Plastination.

Walls, E.W. 1964. "John Bell, 1763–1820." *Medical History* Vol. 8, No. 1 (Jan.): 63–69.

Walter, Tony. 2004a. "Body Worlds: Clinical Detachment and Anatomical Awe." *Sociology of Health and Illness* Vol. 26, No. 4: 464–488.

_____. 2004b. "Plastination for Display: A New Way to Dispose of the Dead." *Journal of the Royal Anthropological Institute* Vol. 10, No. 3 (Sept.).

Warner, John Harley, and James M. Edmonson. 2009. *Dissection: Photographs of a Rite of Passage in American Medicine 1880–1930.* New York: Blast Books.

Washington, Harriet A. 2006. *Medical Apartheid: The Dark History of Medical*

Experimentation on Black Americans from Colonial Times to the Present. New York: Anchor Books.

"The Wax Anatomical Models at the Josephinum." 2007. Curious Expeditions [http://curiousexpeditions.org/?p=19, accessed 8/19/2011].

Wetz, Franz Josef. 2004a. "Modern Anatomical Theater: The First Public Autopsy in 200 Years." In Gunther von Hagens and Angelina Whalley, *Body Worlds: The Anatomical Exhibition of Real Human Bodies.* Heidelberg, Germany: Institute fur Plastination.

―――. 2004b. "The Dignity of Man." In Gunther von Hagens and Angelina Whalley, *Body Worlds: The Anatomical Exhibition of Real Human Bodies.* Heidelberg: Institut für Plastination.

Wilson, Luke. 1987. "William Harvey's *Prelectiones*: The Performance of the Body in the Renaissance Theater of Anatomy." *Representations* No. 17 (Winter): 62–95.

Wise, Sarah. 2004. *The Italian Boy: A Tale of Murder and Body Snatching in 1830s London.* New York: Henry Holt and Co.

Wolfe, S.J., with Robert Singerman. 2009. *Mummies in Nineteenth Century America: Ancient Egyptians as Artifacts.* Jefferson, NC: McFarland.

Zaner, Richard M. 1992. "Parted Bodies, Departed Souls: The Body in Ancient Medicine and Anatomy." In Drew Leder, ed., *The Body in Medical Thought and Practice.* Dordrecht: Kluwer Academic Publishers.

Zwolak, Judith. 1999. "A Tale of Two Mummies." *Tulanian* (Spring) [http://www2.tulane.edu/feature_mummies_1.cfm, accessed 5/18/09].

Index

anatomical waxes 4, 106–109, 125–137
anatomy: cabinets 4; demonstrations 1, 65, 95–97, 110, 116–117, 122–123; education 31, 50, 65, 70–73, 84–85, 88, 145; lectures 1, 58, 59, 67, 74, 82–83, 93, 112; textbooks 66, 95–96, 99–100, 102–104, 123, 158; theaters 3, 18, 36, 48, 82, 97–98, 119, 152–158, 199
Anatomy Act 46–47, 199
anthropodermic books 6, 7, 21–23, 25, 28–29
autopsy 9, 77, 112, 180, 190–196

Baartman, Saartjie 160–166, 198
barber-surgeons 15, 37, 40, 42, 43, 81, 86, 97, 121–122, 149–150, 199
Barnum, P.T. 10, 22, 33, 178–180, 204
Bell, John 19, 98–101
Bentham, Jeremy 29, 56, 181
body 40; donation 1, 15, 47, 56, 74, 84, 188, 200; mutilation 40, 87, 176
bodysnatching 2, 14, 30, 42, 43, 50–58, 71, 85, 86, 167, 197
BodyWorlds *see* plastination
Buonarroti, Michelangelo *see* Michelangelo
burial, denial of 37, 42
Burke, William 4–5, 15, 50, 60–64
Byrne, Charles 56, 69

cadaver: female 75, 80–81, 94, 149, 164–166, 182; identity 87; modeling 127–129, 136–137; nudity 107, 131–132; processing 141–142, 181; public exposure 5; symbolism 17, 113–114, 147–149, 201; *see also* body
camera obscura 123–125
cannibalism 2, 45
Cheselden, William 58, 85, 105, 121–125
Clift, William 39–40
Cooper, Sir Astley 30, 52, 57–58, 70–74, 102, 189

Corder, William 23–25, 29
corpse *see* body; cadaver
Creed, George 24
Cunningham, William 52–55
Cuvier, Georges 20–21, 160–166

da Carpi, Jacopo Berengario 81
Darwin, Charles 60
death masks 24, 28, 44, 63
de Chauliac, Guy 77–79
de Liuzzi, Mondino 6, 13, 75, 79, 90–93, 204
de Sade, Marquis *see* Sade, Marquis de
dissection: in ancient times 76–77; by artists 80, 100; definition 9–11; as entertainment 149–151, 169–174, 178–180, 184–186, 201; legislation 37, 40–41, 46–47, 73, 81–82; as performance 147–149; as punishment 37, 40–41, 62, 64; religious opposition 77–78, 87

embalming 4, 6, 39, 108, 110, 115–116, 140–141, 157, 168, 176; *see also* plastination
execution 15, 23–24, 26, 37, 40, 43, 61–63, 66, 90, 94, 144, 188; survival 42–43; of women 38, 43

Fontana, Felice 126–127
Fragonard, Honoré 4, 6, 30, 31, 108, 138–142, 180–182, 202

Galen 6, 12, 14, 17, 75, 77, 204
gibbeting 37, 38, 41, 42
Gliddon, George Robins 175–176
Gray, Henry 6, 101–104
Grazemark, Richard 144–145

Hare, William 15, 50, 60
Harvey, William 1, 6, 82–83, 148, 199, 203, 204
Hawass, Zahi 177

INDEX

Herophilus 12, 75, 77, 204
Heth, Joice 178–180, 200
Hogarth, William 7, 35–37
Horwood, John 25–26
"Hottentot Venus" *see* Baartman, Saartjie
Hough, John Stockton 22
Howison, John 64 – 65
human leather *see* tanning of human skin
Hunter, John 6, 17, 55–57, 64–70, 71, 81, 167
Hunter, William 65–70, 80, 85

"Irish giant" *see* Byrne, Charles

Joseph II of Austria 129–130

Knox, Robert 60–62, 199

LeBlanc, Antoine 26
Leonardo da Vinci 14, 17, 80

Manzolini, Anna Morandi 137–138
Mata Hari 38–39
Michelangelo 14, 17, 80
Monro primus, Alexander 57–60, 65, 199–200
Monro secundus, Alexander 57, 59–60, 98–99
Monro tertius, Alexander 57, 60, 63–64
mummy "unrolling" 5, 10, 15, 33, 167–178, 189, 200
"Murder in the Red Barn" *see* Corder, William
museum specimens 6, 40, 44, 63, 64, 68–70, 102, 106–108, 116, 126–127, 141–143, 156, 202

"Old Cunny" *see* Cunningham, William

Paaw, Pieter 59
pathology 10, 86
Peter the Great 117–118

Pettigrew, Thomas 7, 166–175
photography 2, 15, 88–89, 101–102, 146–147; *see also* camera obscura
phrenology 24–25, 44
plastination 181–184; *see also* von Hagens, Gunther

Rembrandt van Rijn 14, 75, 119–121, 146, 158–159, 204
"Reward of Cruelty" *see* Hogarth, William
Royal College of Surgeons 35, 42, 43, 83, 102, 125, 170
Ruysch, Fredrick 4, 6, 30, 58, 106, 108, 109–121, 204

Sade, Marquis de 135
Saliceto, William of 77
Shippen, William, Jr. 87
skeletons 6, 20, 26, 28, 35, 39, 44, 55, 59, 70, 105, 113–114, 123–125, 138–139, 155–156, 164–165, 181, 198; *see also* museum specimens
Smith, Southwood 56
spectacle: definition 32–33; dissection 87, 143, 178, 187–189, 196
Spurzheim, Johann Gaspar 25
Susini, Clemente 30, 125–137
Sweeney Todd 44–45

tanning of human skin 5, 21, 28, 38, 63–64, 145, 156
television 16
Towne, Joseph 136–138
Tulp, Nicolaes 6, 158–160, 180, 204

Vesalius, Andreas 3, 7, 17–19, 75, 93–98, 160, 180, 181, 204
von Hagens, Gunther 6, 11, 16, 31–32, 151, 180–196, 202–204

Zumbo, Gaetano Giulio 134–135, 138

www.ingramcontent.com/pod-product-compliance
Ingram Content Group UK Ltd.
Pitfield, Milton Keynes, MK11 3LW, UK
UKHW041954140426
5217IPUK00015B/801